8/03

Migraine in Women

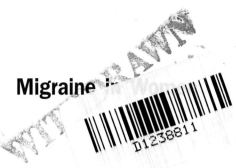

WITHDRAWN

D1238811

Anne MacGregor

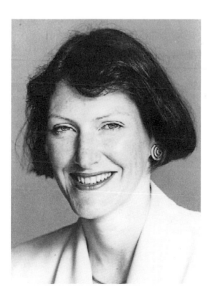

Dr Anne MacGregor qualified from
St Bartholomew's Hospital in 1986. She currently
works at The City of London Migraine Clinic,
London and also in the Department of
Gynaecology, running the Menopause Clinic and
the Sexual Health Clinic as an instructing doctor
in family planning at St Bartholomew's Hospital,
London

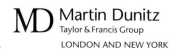 Martin Dunitz
Taylor & Francis Group

LONDON AND NEW YORK

© 2003 Martin Dunitz, an imprint of Taylor & Francis Group

First published in the United Kingdom in 1999
by Martin Dunitz, an imprint of Taylor and Francis Group plc,
11 New Fetter Lane, London EC4P 4EE

Reprinted with revisions 2000
Reprinted with revisions 2003

All rights reserved. No part of this publication may be reproduced, stored in a retrieval system, or transmitted, in any form or by any means, electronic, mechanical, photocopying, recording, or otherwise, without the prior permission of the publisher.

A CIP record for this book is available from the British Library.

ISBN 1 84184 205 2

Distributed in the USA by
Fulfilment Center
Taylor & Francis
10650 Tobben Drive
Independence, KY 41051, USA
Toll Free Tel.: +1 800 634 7064
E-mail: taylorandfrancis@thomsonlearning.com

Distributed in Canada by
Taylor & Francis
74 Rolark Drive
Scarborough, Ontario M1R 4G2, Canada
Toll Free Tel.: +1 877 226 2237
E-mail: tal_fran@istar.ca

Distributed in the rest of the world by
Thomson Publishing Services
Cheriton House
North Way
Andover, Hampshire SP10 5BE, UK
Tel.: +44 (0)1264 332424
E-mail: salesorder.tandf@thomsonpublishingservices.co.uk

Composition by Scribe Design, Gillingham, Kent, UK
Printed and bound in Italy by Printer Trento S.r.l.

Cover illustration from Migraine Art by permission of the Migraine Action Association and Boehringer Ingelheim.

Contents

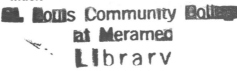

Preface

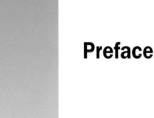

> Migraine is least common in healthy males, restricted to the sexual time of life, occurs after an accumulation of internal or external stimuli, is characterised by periodicity of outbreaks, and results from complex aetiology (Freud, 1895).

Migraine is a condition that has always plagued the human race. It is the subject of numerous myths and misconceptions–including the myths that migraine only affects hysterical women and that it is something sufferers have to learn to live with. Migraine is more common in women during the reproductive years, owing to the additional hormonal triggers. It is now recognized as an organic condition resulting from biochemical changes for which effective treatments are available to help prevent and treat attacks. If standard management strategies are inadequate, much can also be done to lessen and treat the effect of hormonal triggers, as this book shows.

Acknowledgements

I am grateful to Dr Bill Laughey for his comments.

Recommendations for treatment are based on *Guidelines for all Doctors in the Diagnosis and Management of Migraine* available from the British Association for the Study of Headache (see 'Useful Information', p. 79).

Readers are advised to refer to the summary of product characteristics or data sheet for full drug information on contraindications, precautions, drug interactions, and adverse reactions.[1] For updated information, contact the relevant pharmaceutical company as listed in the British National Formulary (BNF) or The Monthly Index of Medical Specialities (MIMS).

[1]ABPI Compendium of Data Sheets and Summaries of Product Characteristics. London: Datapharm Publications Ltd.

What is migraine?

1

Migraine is a benign episodic condition. Headache is usually the main symptom, lasting 4–72 hours, associated with nausea, vomiting, dislike of light, sound, and smells, all of which make it difficult for the person to function normally during an attack. There is complete freedom from symptoms between attacks, so daily headaches are not migraine, although migraine and daily headaches may coexist.

The frequency of attacks is extremely variable with periods of exacerbation and respite, sometimes with frequent migraines for a few months and then none for some time–even several years. Some people experience only one or two attacks during their lifetimes. The average frequency is one to two attacks every one or two months. Attacks more often than once a week are unlikely to be migraine alone and may indicate exacerbation of symptoms as a result of overuse of analgesics or other acute headache medication.

Migraine has an impact on work and social and family life–not only because of inability to function during an attack but also through fear of having an attack. There is no existing cure for migraine and its natural history is not affected by treatment, which seems only to suppress the manifestations of the condition.

Types of migraine

There are two main subtypes of migraine, which may coexist: *migraine without aura* accounts for 70–90% of attacks, and *migraine with aura* accounts for 10–30% of attacks. One to two per cent of attacks are of *migraine aura without headache*. Different types of migraine may coexist. Other types are rarely seen.

The International Headache Society (IHS) has produced a classification of headaches and diagnostic criteria (see page 82). This defines the most important features of migraine.

Migraine without aura (formerly common or simple migraine):

> an idiopathic, recurring headache disorder manifesting in attacks lasting 4–72 hours. Typical characteristics of headache are unilateral location, pulsating quality, moderate or severe intensity, aggravation by routine physical activity, and association with nausea, photo- and phonophobia.

Migraine with aura (formerly classical or focal migraine):

> an idiopathic, recurring disorder manifesting with attacks of neurological symptoms unequivocally localizable to cerebral cortex or brain stem, usually gradually developed over 15–20 minutes and usually lasting less than 60 minutes. Headache, nausea and/or photophobia usually follow the neurological aura symptoms directly or after a free interval of less than an hour. The headache usually lasts 4–72 hours.

The clinical picture of migraine

No definition accurately reflects all the symptoms of migraine; it is much more than just a headache (Figure 1). Based on the clinical picture, the attack can be divided into five distinct stages.

Prodromes

Some migraineurs (or more often their friends or family) recognize warning symptoms of subtle changes in mood or behaviour, up to 24 hours before the headache. This phase can precede attacks of both migraine with aura and migraine without aura:

- Altered mental state–irritability, feeling 'high' or 'low'; some patients describe feeling 'dangerously' well.
- Altered behaviour–hyperactivity, or clumsiness and extreme lethargy.
- Altered appearance–pale, sunken eyes.
- Neurological symptoms–tired or yawning, dysphasia, photo- and phono-phobia, generalized blurred vision.
- Muscular aches and pains.

- Alimentary symptoms–craving for foods, anorexia, constipation; craving for sweet foods may result in a desire to eat chocolate or other sweets which are incorrectly blamed as a cause of the attack.
- Symptoms related to fluid balance–increased urinary frequency, thirst or fluid retention.

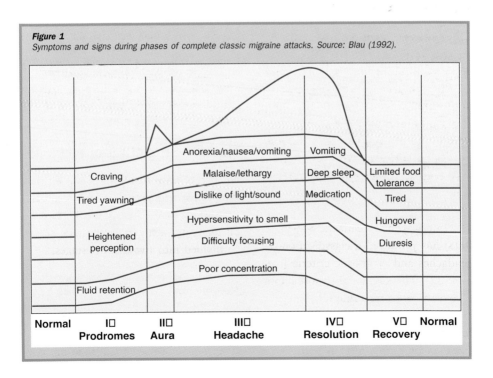

Figure 1
Symptoms and signs during phases of complete classic migraine attacks. Source: Blau (1992).

Aura

Specific focal neurological symptoms of migraine aura last up to an hour (typically 20–30 minutes), usually resolving before the headache starts. There may be a gap of up to an hour between the end of the aura and the start of the headache. Visual symptoms nearly always occur. These are usually symmetrical, affecting one hemifield of both eyes, although subjectively they often appear to affect only one eye. Initially the patient barely notices a small bright spot in the visual field, which becomes more apparent as it begins to expand into a 'C' or inverted 'C' shape, shimmering with zigzags at the edges. This continues to travel across the visual field, eventually breaking up and disappearing. Occasionally, sensory symptoms occur in conjuction with visual aura. A sensation of pins and needles, usually affecting one arm, typically travels up from the hand over several minutes to affect the face and tongue.

Headache

This can be severe and throbbing, particularly in attacks of migraine without aura. It is often, but not necessarily, unilateral. The sufferer usually feels nauseous, and may vomit, is sensitive to light and sound, and feels generally very weak and unwell. Most have to sit or lie down with the curtains drawn, keeping still, as movement aggravates the pain and nausea. The headache usually lasts for a day, but can last up to three days.

Resolution

Sleep and food aid the resolution of both treated and untreated migraine attacks.

Recovery

After the headache has gone, many migraineurs feel drained for a further day, although some are elated with the relief that the attack has passed. In-between attacks, they feel completely well, free from migraine symptoms.

Key points

- Migraine is characterized by episodic attacks of headache with associated nausea, photophobia, and general malaise, lasting 4–72 hours with complete freedom from symptoms between attacks.
- Some migraine headaches are preceded by focal neurological symptoms of aura.

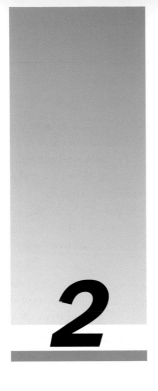

Who gets migraine and why?

Migraine is common, affecting both sexes. Onset is typically during childhood or adolescence (Figure 2). A first attack after age 50 is unusual and warrants further investigation. Epidemiological studies suggest that, before puberty, boys and girls

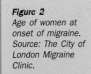

Figure 2
Age of women at onset of migraine. Source: The City of London Migraine Clinic.

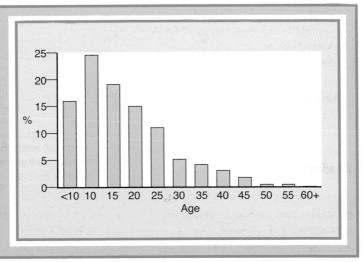

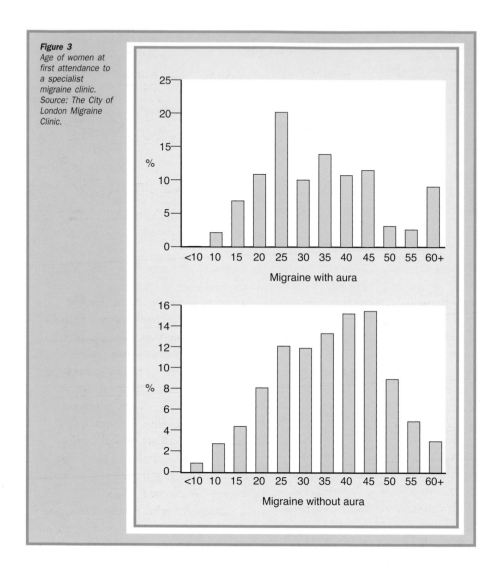

Figure 3
*Age of women at
first attendance to
a specialist
migraine clinic.
Source: The City of
London Migraine
Clinic.*

are equally affected with approximately 6% of 7-year-olds reporting
migraine. After puberty prevalence,

particularly of migraine without aura,
increases to peak during the early 40s
(Figure 3). During the reproductive

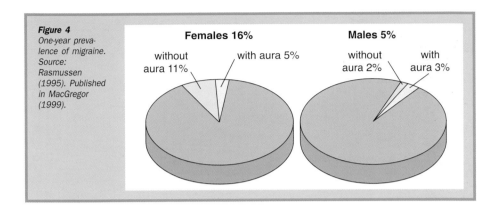

Figure 4
*One-year preva-
lence of migraine.
Source:
Rasmussen
(1995). Published
in MacGregor
(1999).*

years there are marked gender differences in the prevalence and type of
migraine, with migraine without aura
affecting more women (Figure 4). In
both sexes, migraine typically improves
after age 55.

Migraine triggers

Many varied triggers can provoke
migraine (Figure 5). Women are also
affected by female sex hormones,
which can have profound effects on
the frequency, severity, and type of
migraine–both good and bad. This
additional hormonal trigger may
account for the increased prevalence in
migraine in women compared with
men during the reproductive years.

Triggers appear to be cumulative,
reaching a threshold above which the
biochemical process of migraine is
initiated (Figure 6). Hence, non-
hormonal factors are still important,
even when there appears to be a
strong link between the hormonal
cycle and migraine. For example,
triggers accumulate over the month,
such as disturbed sleep and muscle
tension, resulting from stress at work
or at home, missed meals, etc.
Combine this with menstruation, and
an attack ensues. All these triggers are
equally important–stress, lack of sleep,
muscle tension, lack of food, and
hormones. Dealing with any of these
triggers may reduce the likelihood of
an attack.

Figure 5
Trigger factors for migraine.

Insufficient food
- Missing meals
- Delayed meals
- Inadequate quantity

Specific foods
- Occasionally cheese, chocolate, citrus fruits (but cravings may be prodromal symptoms)
- Certain wines/beers/spirits
- Caffeine withdrawal

Sleep
- Oversleeping
- Lack of sleep

Head and neck pains
- Eyes, sinuses, neck, teeth, or jaw pain

Emotional triggers

Environmental
- Bright or flickering lights
- Overexertion/exercise
- Travel
- Weather changes
- Strong smells

Hormonal factors (women)
- Menstruation
- Oral contraception
- Pregnancy (may exacerbate focal symptoms but usually migraine improves in the second and third trimesters)
- HRT

Intercurrent illness

Note: Not all the above apply to every migraine patient and usually more than one factor has to be present to initiate an attack.

Figure 6
'Threshold' theory of migraine.
Source: MacGregor (1996).

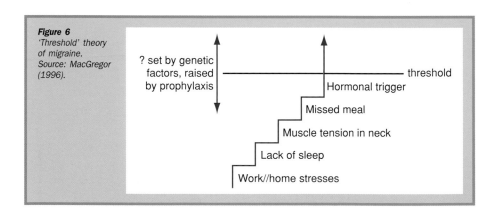

? set by genetic factors, raised by prophylaxis

threshold

Hormonal trigger

Missed meal

Muscle tension in neck

Lack of sleep

Work//home stresses

Key points

- Migraine is common.
- Migraine starts in the young, is at peak prevalence during the reproductive years, and improves in both sexes in later life.
- Migraine affects three times as many women as men.
- Sex hormones have varying effects on the frequency, severity, and type of migraine.
- Non-hormonal triggers should be identified, even when a strong hormonal link with migraine is apparent.

Clinical diagnosis

3

Taking a careful history is crucial, as the diagnosis of migraine rests solely on the history. The physical examination is essentially normal and there are no confirmatory diagnostic tests or investigations currently available.

History

It is usually possible to make the diagnosis in the first few minutes of the consultation. If the history is confusing, consider if there is more than one type of headache present by asking the patient 'How many different headaches do you have?' and taking a separate history for each headache. At the very least, the following questions should be used. More extensive questioning is necessary if there is any uncertainty or suspicion of the presence of a more serious underlying disorder:

• *Can you describe a typical attack?*
Most patients with migraine describe
a one-sided throbbing headache with
nausea and/or vomiting, photophobia,
and phonophobia, which may be
preceded by prodromal symptoms
and/or aura. Effective medication,
sleep, and vomiting usually resolve
symptoms. Although open-ended
questions are best, symptoms can be
elicited by asking: 'Can you tell when
you are going to get an attack before
the headache starts?' 'Do you notice
any weakness or numbness?' 'Do you
have any problems with your speech
or vision?', 'Does light, sound, or
smell bother you?' 'Do you feel sick
or are you sick?' 'How does an attack
end?'
• *What do you do when you have an
attack?* Some migraineurs manage to
struggle through the day and collapse
in bed when they get home. Others
cannot get to work or have to leave
work early. They typically retire to bed
in a quiet, darkened room and try to
lie still since movement can aggravate
pain and nausea.
• *What do the headaches stop you
doing?* Frequent attacks can result in
severe disability during an attack as
well as through fear of an impending
attack. Such situations warrant more
aggressive management than mild,
infrequent migraine.
• *How old were you when you had your
first attack?* Migraine starts in the
young; it is unusual for a first attack

to occur in a patient over 55 years.
However, the older patient may seek
help for exacerbation of migraine after
several years of respite. If there is
any doubt, the older patient should be
investigated further.
• *How do you feel in-between attacks?*
Most patients answer 'Fine'. If the
patient has symptoms between
attacks, look for additional headaches
or other pathology.
• *How often do you have an attack?*
Migraine is an episodic condition. If
the patient complains of daily or near
daily headaches, then the diagnosis
of the primary headache is unlikely to
be migraine. However, patients may
have had attacks of migraine for
many years which they have
controlled, but daily headaches are
the reason why they have sought
help, particularly if the superimposed
migraine attacks have also become
more frequent and less responsive to
treatment.
• *How long does the attack last?* Most
attacks last for part of a day, and up
to three days.
• *What do you take when you have an
attack?* Check whether or not the
patient takes appropriate medication
early enough and in an adequate
dose. Inquire about past drug and
non-drug treatments as these may be
worth trying again if they were not
used optimally. A full drug history is
essential to exclude medication-
misuse headache (see below).

Examination

A general physical and a neurological examination are essential, with particular emphasis placed on the relevant systems. The examination must be complete but can be brief. At the very least, fundoscopy should be performed to ensure there is no evidence of raised intracranial pressure. Blood pressure should also be measured as, although hypertension is rarely a cause of headache, most patients think it is.

Investigations

No investigations can confirm the diagnosis of migraine–they should be used only to exclude secondary causes of headache.

Useful aids: diary cards

Diary cards can aid diagnosis of migraine and other headaches, especially if several coexist. Patients should be asked to record all their attacks on the diary card, noting the following information as a minimum:

1) Date.
2) Day of the week.
3) Time the attack started.
4) Symptoms present and how they changed.
5) How long the attack lasted.
6) What treatment was taken.
7) What time it was taken.
8) How effective treatment was.
9) How the attack ended.

A record of migraine will show attacks occurring episodically with days in between when the patient is headache free. Symptoms of non-migraine headache may also be apparent (see below). A pattern of attacks may be obvious (days of the week, time of day), revealing potential triggers (sleeping late at weekends, missed meals, etc.). Use of acute drugs can be checked for optimal dosing. Frequent use of acute medication should alert the doctor to medication misuse.

How does migraine differ from other common headaches?

Most non-migraine headaches are easy to diagnose from their typical presentation.

Tension headache

A continuous headache, often described as a band around, or a weight on top of, the head. It lasts throughout the day, rarely interferes with daily activities, and is unaffected by analgesics. It is often associated with underlying depression. Antidepressants such as amitriptyline are usually effective.

Muscle contraction headache

Conditions such as cervical spondylosis and temporomandibular joint dysfunction can give rise to local muscle pain. The affected muscle(s) are often tender to touch. Analgesics help, usually within about 30 minutes. For long-term control, physical treatments, including physiotherapy or acupuncture, are recommended since drugs only provide short-term relief.

Medication-misuse headaches

The existence of headaches related to the overuse of ergotamine has been recognized for many years; more recently exacerbation of headache associated with the overconsumption of any acute drugs has been identified. Anyone taking acute drugs to treat headache regularly on more than three days a week is at risk. The patient will complain of frequent headache or

'daily' migraine, with only limited response to treatment. The only effective treatment is to stop the medication as the headache is refractory to drug or non-drug prophylaxis.

Is it something more serious?

Recent headaches can result from underlying pathology affecting the ears (otitis media), the nasopharynx (nasopharyngeal carcinoma), sinuses (sinusitis), eyes (glaucoma), teeth (impacted wisdom teeth), temporomandibular joints, upper cervical spine, and temporal arteries.

Is it a brain tumour?

Patients (and doctors) often fear the presence of a brain tumour but these rarely present with symptoms of headache alone. The tumour infiltrates the tissues of the brain and usually produces focal neurological symptoms and signs, and occasionally epilepsy, in addition to a headache, classically worse on waking, and associated with vomiting. Symptoms progress as the tumour enlarges. The history is usually sufficient to make the diagnosis (Table 1) and prompts a thorough physical examination which usually reveals abnormal signs.

Table 1
Differences between a cerebral tumour and migraine.

	Tumour	**Migraine**
History	Months	Years
Attack frequency	Usually progressive	Intermittent
Pain	Deep, steady, dull ache	Throbbing
Site of pain	Unilateral and always in the same place	Variable
Vomiting	Spontaneous and does not relieve headache	Associated with nausea and often relieves headache
Effect of movement/ coughing/straining	Aggravates headache	Aggravates headache
Onset of symptoms	Wakes patient from sleep	Present on waking or develops during the day

Is it an aura or a transient ischaemic attack?

The concern about aura or a transient ischaemic attack (TIA) (Table 2) is particularly important for women taking combined oral contraceptives. Fortunately, there are distinguishing differences between the focal neurological symptoms of migraine aura and a TIA or ischaemic stroke.

In essence, symptoms of migraine aura are typically progressive and positive compared to the sudden onset of negative symptoms suggestive of an ischaemic event.

Key points

- Migraine diagnosis is based on a history of typical symptoms in the absence of physical signs.
- No diagnostic tests or investigations are available to confirm the diagnosis and should only be used if secondary headaches are considered.
- Daily headaches are not migraine but may coexist with migraine.
- Medication-misuse headache should be considered in patients with frequent headaches, using acute treatments regularly more often than three days each week.
- Diary cards are an invaluable aid to diagnosis and management.

Table 2
Difference between ischaemic episodes and migraine aura.

	TIA	Migraine
History	No previous episodes	Similar attacks in the past (typically migraine onset childhood/early adulthood)
Onset/progression of symptoms	Sudden (seconds)	Slow evolution over several minutes
Duration	> 1 hour	< 1 hour (typically 20–30 minutes)
Timing	Occurs with or without headache, with no temporal relationship	Precedes and resolves before onset of typical migraine headache
Visual symptoms	Monocular, negative (black) scotoma	99% auras; homonymous positive (bright) scotoma gradually enlarging across visual field into 'C' shape with scintillating zigzag edges
Sensory/motor symptoms	May occur without visual symptoms May include leg Negative (limb feels 'dead')	One-third auras–usually in association with visual symptoms Rarely affects leg Positive ('pins and needles')
Headache	No subsequent headache or symptoms continue in association with headache	Migraine headache and associated symptoms typically follow resolution of aura. Aura may occur without headache, but confirm past history of migraine

Managing migraine: an overview

4

Effective management of migraine is dependent on correct diagnosis. If migraine coexists with other headaches, non-migraine headaches should be treated first as this may in itself reduce the frequency and severity of migraine (Figure 7).

For infrequent attacks, acute therapy may suffice. Prophylaxis is indicated for frequent attacks or when acute treatment alone is inadequate.

For most women, standard acute and prophylactic treatments suffice. When there is an obvious hormonal trigger, evidenced by diary cards, consider more specific management regimens as discussed in the appropriate sections. However, it should be noted that hormonal therapies are rarely indicated as most attacks respond to the more conservative initial approaches outlined.

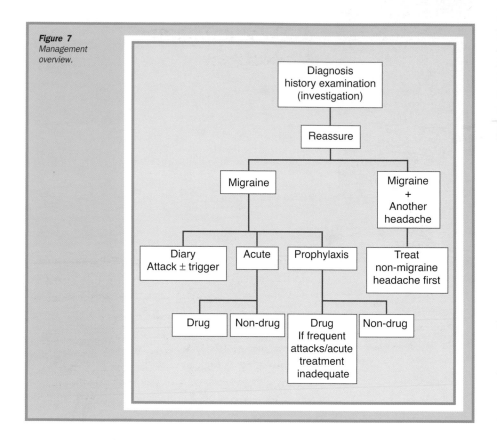

*Management
overview.*

Acute treatment

5

Acute treatments are used to abort or reduce symptoms once an attack has started. Since attacks vary in frequency and severity, even in the same patient, a treatment ladder is suggested.

Patients start at the lowest rung of the ladder they think will be effective for each attack. If they recognize mild symptoms early they should start with step one. If this proves ineffective after one hour, or symptoms are severe at the onset, they may treat from the second stage. If, after three attacks, the first stage is always ineffective, they should initiate treatment from a higher stage (Figure 8).

If nothing works, review the diagnosis. Some patients become refractory to therapy when they overuse acute medication. This should be considered for patients who do not respond to treatment and who have regularly been using acute headache treatments on more than 3 days each week.

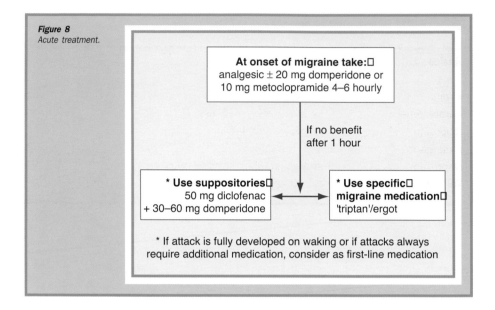

Figure 8
Acute treatment.

At onset of migraine take:
analgesic ± 20 mg domperidone or
10 mg metoclopramide 4–6 hourly

If no benefit
after 1 hour

* **Use suppositories**
50 mg diclofenac
+ 30–60 mg domperidone

* **Use specific**
migraine medication
'triptan'/ergot

* If attack is fully developed on waking or if attacks always
require additional medication, consider as first-line medication

Step 1: oral analgesics with or without domperidone or metoclopramide

Simple oral analgesics such as aspirin, ibuprofen or paracetamol, preferably soluble, may be effective if taken early in an attack, in adequate doses. Non-steroidal anti-inflammatory drugs (NSAIDs) such as diclofenac, naproxen, and tolfenamic acid may also be tried early in an attack and are particularly useful when tenderness in the scalp or neck muscles is a prominent symptom (Table 3). Aspirin is contraindicated in children under the age of 12. Patients with gastrointestinal ulceration, gout, or bleeding disorders should avoid NSAIDs. Specific over-the-counter analgesic combinations, some of which contain antiemetics, are also available and popular with some patients.

Absorption may be improved with prokinetic antiemetic drugs, as migraine is associated with gastrointestinal stasis and reduced rate of gastric emptying. Domperidone and metoclopramide are the drugs of choice and should be used even when patients are not nauseous in

Table 3
Analgesics.

Analgesic	Dose (mg)
Aspirin	600–900 every 4–6 hrs
Paracetamol	500–1000 every 4–6 hrs
Ibuprofen	400–800 every 4–6 hrs
Diclofenac	Oral and rectal: 50 every 8–12 hrs
Naproxen	Oral and rectal: 250–500 every 12 hrs
Tolfenamic acid	Oral: 200 repeat once after 2–3 hrs if necessary

Table 4
Prokinetic antiemetics.

Antiemetic	Dose (mg)
Domperidone	Oral: 20 every 4–8 hrs Rectal: 30–60 every 4–8 hrs
Metoclopramide	10 mg every 8 hrs

order to improve the efficacy of analgesics (Table 4). Metoclopramide may cause drowsiness and its use can be associated with acute extrapyramidal reactions in children and young women. Domperidone does not readily cross the blood–brain barrier so side-effects are rarely seen with episodic use.

Step 2: rectal analgesics with or without rectal domperidone

The use of suppositories allows similar drugs to be given, bypassing the gut. Diclofenac suppositories (50 mg) plus domperidone (30–60 mg) every 8 hours are suggested.

Step 3: triptans

These drugs have vasoconstrictor properties; they are not analgesic. There are currently six triptans available: almotriptan, eletriptan, naratriptan, rizatriptan, sumatriptan, and zolmitriptan (Table 5). Although efficacy at 4 hours is similar for all oral preparations, there are several differences, which may make a particular triptan more appropriate for certain patients. Oral almotriptan 12.5 mg offers comparable all round efficacy and tolerability. Oral eletriptan 40 mg has fast onset to efficacy. Oral naratriptan 2.5 mg is slowest to onset of efficacy but has fewest associated side-effects. Oral rizatriptan 10 mg has fastest onset to efficacy; lyophilisate

Table 5
Triptans.

Triptan	Dose (mg)*	Max/24 hours(mg)*
Almotriptan**		
Oral tablet	12.5	25
Eletriptan**		
Oral tablet	20–40	80
Naratriptan**		
Oral tablet	2.5	5
Sumatriptan**		
Oral tablet	50–100	300
Intranasal	20	40
Subcutaneous	6	12
Suppository (not UK)	25	50
Rizatriptan**		
Oral tablet	5–10	20
Oral lyophilisate (wafer)	10	20
Zolmitriptan***		
Oral tablet	2.5–5	10
Orodispersible tablet	2.5–5	10
Intranasal	5	10

* *Doses as recommended in the UK at the time of writing. Always refer to local prescribing guidelines.*
** *Repeat dose once in 24 hours for recurrence only after initial response.*
*** *Repeat dose 2 hours after initial dose for lack of effect or recurrence.*

(wafer) rizatriptan 10 mg melts on the tongue and is useful if liquids are not available. However, onset to effect is slower than with the tablet. Oral zolmitriptan 2.5 mg has better dosing flexibility than the other available triptans, as a second dose can be taken 2 hours after lack of response to the initial dose. A 5 mg initial dose can be taken if a second dose has always been necessary at 2 hours. A mouth-dispersable preparation (Rapimelt®) and fast-acting nasal spray are also available.

Oral sumatriptan 50 mg should be continued if a patient is established on it and satisfied. Oral sumatriptan 100 mg is a second-line triptan if a more potent drug is required.

If vomiting precludes oral therapy, subcutaneous sumatriptan should be used. For rapid onset, consider intra-nasal and subcutaneous sumatriptan.

Adverse events typical to triptans include dizziness, somnolence, asthenia, and nausea. 'Chest' symptoms, including tightness and pressure in the throat, neck, and chest, are more common with sumatriptan than the other triptans. The concern that such symptoms are of cardiac origin is not confirmed by ECG studies, which rarely show changes suggestive of ischaemia. However, the cause of 'chest' symptoms remains unclear and caution is indicated.

Contraindications to triptans include any condition associated with risk of stroke or coronary artery disease, uncontrolled hypertension, ischaemic heart disease, and concomitant use of ergotamine or other 5-HT$_1$ agonists. Triptans are not recommended for elderly patients, even when apparently asymptomatic of vascular disease. There are no clinically relevant inter-actions between almotriptan and standard migraine prophylactic drugs but caution is indicated when prescrib-ing almotriptan to patients with known hypersensitivity to sulphonamides. Eletriptan should not be used together with potent CYP3A4 inhibitors e.g. ketoconazole, itraconi-zole, erythromycine, clarithromycin, josamycin, and protease inhibitors (ritonavir, indinavir and nelfinavir). Sumatriptan should not be used concomitantly with monoamine oxidase inhibitors (MAOIs), selective 5HT reuptake inhibitors (SSRIs), or lithium. Naratriptan should not be used concomitantly with methysergide. Caution should be exercised before using sumatriptan or naratriptan in patients with known hypersensitivity to sulphonamides. Rizatriptan should not be used concomitantly with MAOIs and there is a theoretical interaction with SSRIs and CYP2DG substrates. The 5 mg dose is recommended for patients taking propranolol. Zolmitriptan should not be used in patients with Wolff–Parkinson–White syndrome or arrhythmias asssociated with other accessory pathways. The maximum daily dose of zolmitriptan should be limited to 7.5 mg in patients taking moclobemide (5 mg in other European countries than the UK) and 5 mg in patients taking cimetidine.

Recurrence of symptoms

A clinical problem identified with triptan use is recurrence of symptoms after initial response, typically within 12–24 hours. This can occur on several consecutive days and is distressing to some patients. A second dose of the same triptan is usually effective but may not be the most appropriate treatment, particularly for repeated recurrence. Instead oral or rectal diclofenac may be tried. If recurrence is a continuing problem, ergots (with a longer half-life) may be more appropriate than triptans.

Table 6
Ergotamine.

Route	Dose	Max dose/week*
Oral	1–2 mg	2
Rectal	1–2 mg (half to one suppository)	2

* Author's recommendation.

Migril (Glaxo Wellcome) = ergotamine tartrate 2 mg, cyclizine hydrochloride 50 mg, caffeine 100 mg.

Cafergot (Sandoz) = ergotamine tartrate 1 mg, caffeine 100 mg.

Cafergot (Sandoz) - ergotamine tartrate 2 mg, caffeine 100 mg.

Step 4: ergots

Ergotamine (Table 6) rectally (1 mg = half a Cafergot® suppository) is the preferred route of delivery. Oral ergotamine has very poor and variable bioavailability and is not recommended. Ergotamine has a narrow therapeutic window so the dose should be titrated against symptoms, starting with a low dose. Side-effects include nausea, vomiting, cold peripheries, muscle aches, and general malaise. Patients should also be counselled about misuse, which can result in daily headache or even ergotism with thrombosis and gangrene. Ideally, treatment should not be repeated after the initial dose, and should not be used again within 4 days. Contraindications to use are similar to the triptans. Concomitant use of beta-blockers should be avoided. Ergots should not be used if the attack has already been treated with a triptan or dihydroergotamine, and vice versa.

Dihydroergotamine (Table 7) has fewer adverse effects than ergotamine. In those countries where it is available, 1 metered dose of the nasal spray should be used in each nostril (i.e. a total of 2 doses) at the onset of an attack. An additional 1–2 doses can be repeated after a minimum of 15 minutes for lack of response. Treatment may be repeated after an interval of 8 hours to a maximum of 8 metered doses in 24 hours. Side-effects specific to the intranasal route include bad taste and local nasal symptoms such as rhinitis, stuffy nose, and flushing. Other reactions include nausea and vomiting, numbness and tingling in fingers and

Table 7
Dihydroergotamine.

Route	Dose	Max dose/week*
Intranasal	1–2 × 2 mg metered doses	8 metered doses

* Author's recommendation.

toes, and chest tightness. Contraindications are similar to the triptans. Concomitant use of macrolide antibiotics such as erythromycin should be avoided since they may increase the plasma level of dihydroergotamine. Patients susceptible to vasoconstriction should avoid concomitant beta-blockers.

How to make drugs more effective

Oral therapy is usually less effective if taken too late since gastric stasis can develop, inhibiting drug absorption. Secondly, the efficacy of a drug is limited and if the level of pain exceeds the analgesic activity of the drug, stronger medication becomes necessary. Patients should be advised to carry at least a single dose of their preferred medication so that they can take it as soon as they feel an attack coming on.

Sleep can aid recovery; struggling on through the migraine usually only prolongs the attack. Other simple measures can be surprisingly effective. For example, alternating the application of a hot-water bottle or heat pad with cold compresses can help relieve pain.

Emergency treatment

When you are called out to a patient with migraine it is important to confirm the diagnosis before treating. Careful handling is necessary as some patients call because they do not believe the doctor takes their migraine seriously. Avoid the use of opioid drugs as they can exacerbate symptoms and have the potential to lead to dependency, particularly for the few patients who then label themselves as unresponsive to more simple management strategies. Diclofenac and domperidone suppositories are the first choice, otherwise intramuscular dicolfenac (75 mg), intramuscular chlorpromazine (25–50 mg) or intramuscular metoclopramide (5–10 mg) may be tried.

Key points

- Provide patients with a selection of treatment for varying severity of attacks.
- If nothing works, review the diagnosis, considering the coexistence of other headache, particularly medication misuse.

Prophylactic treatment

6

The clinical course of migraine is such that periods of exacerbation tend to resolve spontaneously without intervention. No prophylactic drug provides more than 50% improvement—as effective as identification and avoidance of trigger factors. Therefore, trigger factors should always be considered first (see the chapter: 'Who gets migraine and why?'). If prophylactic drugs are prescribed, their continued need should be assessed at each follow-up visit.

Identify triggers

If patients have frequent attacks of migraine, more than once a month, they may find keeping a trigger diary useful, in addition to the attack diary.

The trigger diary

Rather than 'What triggers an attack?', a more useful question is 'How many triggers initiate an attack?' Even the patient's usual daily routine can include triggers she is not aware of because she remains below the threshold of an attack until a few extra triggers crop up. Therefore, it is important to keep a record of potential triggers every day.

Patients should look at the list of common triggers every day, just before they go to bed. They should make a note of any triggers that were present that day, such as shopping or a delayed meal, etc.–even when they do not have a migraine. Women should keep a record of their menstrual periods and any premenstrual symptoms, as well as any regular medication, including the oral contraceptive pill or hormone replacement therapy (HRT).

Treat triggers

The trigger and attack diaries should be reviewed after at least three attacks. Compare the information in each, looking for a build-up of triggers coinciding with the attacks.

Look at the timing of attacks. If they occur early in the morning, late morning, or late afternoon, they may be due to low blood sugar. Eating a snack at bedtime, mid-morning, or

mid-afternoon may be the only treatment necessary to prevent attacks. Note a link with sleeping in at weekends, or with exercise.

Ask the patient to study the list of triggers and divide them into two groups–those the patient can do something about (e.g. missing meals, alcohol) and those which are out of the patient's control (e.g. menstrual cycle, travelling). They should first try to deal with the triggers they have some influence over, cutting out suspect triggers one at a time. Simple advice is to balance triggers–if they are having a particularly stressful time, they should take extra care to eat regularly and find ways to unwind before bedtime.

Although insufficient food is probably the most important dietary trigger, certain foods, in particular cheese, chocolate, alcohol, citrus fruits, dairy produce, and many others, have been implicated. Because several factors are necessary to trigger an attack it follows that if other factors can be identified and minimized, then food triggers will be less important. However, if the patient suspects that a particular food does trigger an attack, that food should be avoided for a few weeks before it is reintroduced. If a large number of foods are involved, consider referral to a dietician as elimination diets run the risk of causing malnutrition if they are not adequately supervised.

Some prodromal symptoms are incorrectly blamed as triggers for the attack. A craving for sweet foods may result in a desire to eat chocolate or other sweet foods. A few people feel 'on top of the world' before an attack and rush around thinking later that the attack was caused by overactivity. These are signs the attack has already begun.

Other measures

Other non-drug measures (including behavioural therapy–consisting of psychological support, relaxation exercises, and biofeedback training) have also been shown to reduce the frequency and severity of migraine.

Drug prophylaxis

The object of prophylaxis is to reduce the frequency and severity of attacks (Table 8). Drugs can usually be withdrawn gradually after 4–6 months. The lowest possible initial

Table 8
Prophylactic drugs.

Drug	Starting dose (mg)	Max daily (mg)
Beta-blocker (e.g. propranolol)	10 twice daily	240 in three divided doses (long-acting once daily)
Amitriptyline*	10 nocte	75 nocte
Pizotifen	0.5 nocte	3 nocte
Sodium valproate*	200 twice daily	1000 in divided doses
Methysergide	1 nocte	2 three times daily

* *Not licensed for migraine in the UK.*

dose is recommended which should be gradually increased at 2–4-week intervals until symptoms are controlled or side-effects limit use. Compliance is poor with more than once or twice daily dosing. The choice of drug usually depends on the presence of concomitant disorders.

First line

Beta-adrenergic blockers are particularly useful if there is associated hypertension or anxiety. Atenolol, metoprolol, nadolol, propranolol, and timolol have all shown efficacy in clinical trials although atenolol is not licensed for migraine in the UK. Typical side-effects include lethargy, vivid dreams, and cold extremities. Patients with asthma, brittle diabetes, chronic obstructive airways disease, myocardial insufficiency, and peripheral vascular disease should avoid beta-blockers. They should not be used concomitantly with ergotamine.

Amitriptyline is particularly useful if there is associated depression, sleep disturbance, or tension-type headache. Higher doses are usually only necessary for associated depression. Most side-effects, including sedation, dry mouth, dizziness, and blurred vision, improve after the initial weeks of treatment. Amitriptyline is contraindicated in myocardial infarction, heart block, and closed-angle glaucoma. Concomitant use of MAOIs (with or within 14 days), other antidepressives, carbamazepine, phenytoin, and alcohol should be avoided.

Pizotifen is particularly useful if poor sleep or poor appetite are also a problem. Daytime doses should be avoided, as sedation is a common side-effect. Caution is indicated in patients with glaucoma or urinary retention. Avoid using in obese patients because of increased appetite.

Sodium valproate has undergone controlled clinical trials and may be useful for additional tension-type headache. It may be necessary to check liver function and clotting before prescribing valproate. Side-effects include weight gain, hair loss, gastrointestinal disturbance, and bruising. Avoid prescribing for patients with hepatic disease or thrombocytopenia. It can enhance the effect of aspirin. Effective contraception is necessary for women taking valproate as fetal abnormalities are common.

Second line

Methysergide should be restricted for severe cases which have failed to respond to alternative therapies owing to the rare possibility of developing retroperitoneal, heart valve, and pleural fibrosis. This is unlikely to occur if the patient stops therapy for at least 1 month after each 6 months of use, gradually reducing the dose during the previous 2–3 weeks. An initial dose of 1 mg daily can be increased by 1 mg every 3 days until response is achieved or to maximum 2 mg three times daily. Side-effects include nausea, dyspepsia, leg cramps, dizziness, and sedation. It should not be used by patients with peripheral vascular disease, severe hypertension, cardiac disease, or impaired hepatic or renal function. Concomitant ergots should be avoided.

Other drugs used for prophylaxis

Calcium channel antagonists such as flunarizine, although widely used in some countries, are of doubtful value. They are not licensed for migraine in the UK.

Clonidine is a centrally acting alpha-adrenoceptor agonist indicated for hypertension, which has shown limited efficacy for migraine prophylaxis. It may have a place in the management of menopausal women with migraine and hot flushes who do not wish to take HRT.

Cyproheptadine is an antihistamine with antiserotonin properties occasionally used in migraine. Side-effects include sedation, weight gain, dry mouth, and dizziness.

Gabapentin is an antiepileptic drug also used for the control of chronic pain conditions. It may be helpful for women whose migraine has worsened around the menopause.

Topiramate is an antiepileptic drug that has shown clinical efficacy for migraine. Although the effective dose has yet to be established, clinical trials suggest a starting dose of 25mg per day increasing by 25mg per week to 200mg per day or the maximum tolerated dose.

Key points

- Identification and avoidance of trigger factors can be as effective as drug prophylaxis.
- Compliance is best with once- or twice-daily doses.
- The continuing need for drug prophylaxis should be repeatedly assessed and is rarely necessary for longer than 4–6 months.

Migraine and menstruation

7

More than 50% of women report that menstruation is a migraine trigger (Figure 9). For most women the association is inconsistent, or they have several attacks throughout the cycle. True 'menstrual' migraine defined as 'attacks of migraine without aura that occur regularly on day 1 of menstruation ± 2 days and at no other time' affects fewer than 10% of women.

Mechanisms

Studies have not identified any consistent biochemical or hormonal abnormalities in women with menstrual migraine, compared with control groups and numerous theoretical mechanisms have been proposed:

'Menstrual' migraine: theories of migraine pathophysiology:

- low progesterone levels
- high progesterone levels
- low oestrogen levels
- high oestrogen levels
- falling oestrogen levels
- high oestrogen/progesterone ratio
- low prolactin levels
- high prolactin reserve
- opioid dysregulation
- disordered sympathetic activity
- impaired carbohydrate tolerance
- response to prostaglandin release
- platelet dysfunction
- magnesium deficiency
- vitamin deficiencies
- inherited immune pattern

One reason may be the wide variation of definitions used in the past for 'menstrual' migraine (Figure 10).

The menstrual cycle is the result of complex positive and negative feedback within the

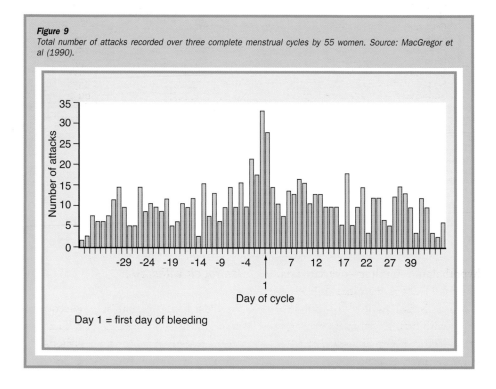

Figure 9
Total number of attacks recorded over three complete menstrual cycles by 55 women. Source: MacGregor et al (1990).

Day 1 = first day of bleeding

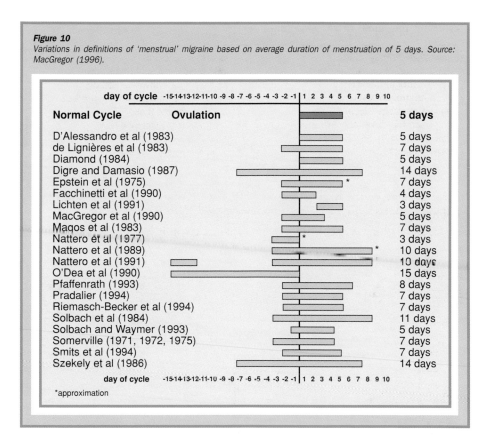

Figure 10
Variations in definitions of 'menstrual' migraine based on average duration of menstruation of 5 days. Source: MacGregor (1996).

hypothalamic–pituitary–ovarian axis (Figure 11). It is therefore unlikely that migraine is the result of any single event within this system. However, two specific events are relevant to migraine management.

Oestrogen withdrawal

The most likely mechanism to account for perimenstrual migraine is falling levels of oestrogen following prolonged oestrogen exposure, such as occurs

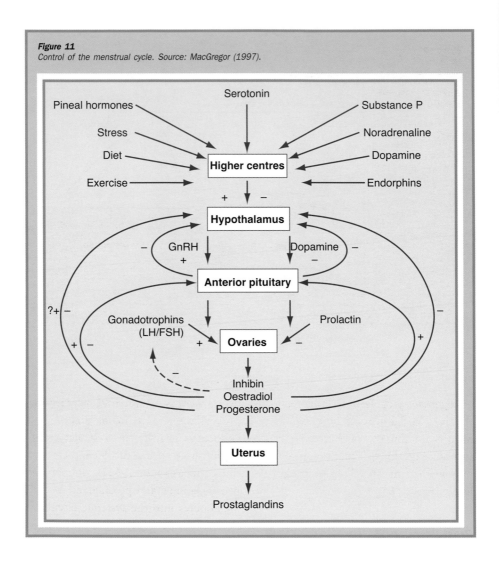

Figure 11
Control of the menstrual cycle. Source: MacGregor (1997).

during the late luteal phase of the normal menstrual cycle (Figure 12). Somerville showed that migraine could be postponed by maintaining high plasma oestradiol levels, despite normal menstruation occurring as

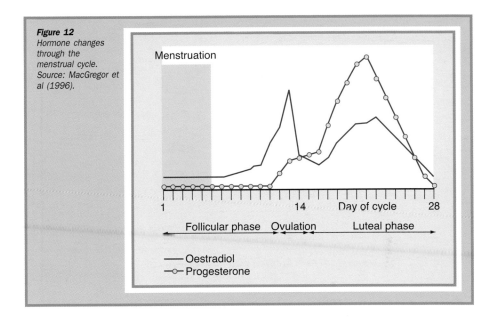

Figure 12
Hormone changes through the menstrual cycle. Source: MacGregor et al (1996).

endogenous progesterone levels fell (Figure 13). He repeated the experiment maintaining progesterone levels. In both experiments, migraine occurred only at the time of falling oestradiol levels (Figure 14).

Prostaglandin release

Entry of prostaglandins into the systemic circulation can trigger throbbing headache, nausea, and vomiting. With regard to the menstrual cycle, there is a three-fold increase in prostaglandin levels in the uterine endometrium from the follicular to the luteal phase with a further increase during menstruation. Maximal entry of prostaglandins and prostaglandin metabolites into the systemic circulation occurs during the first 48 hours of menstruation. This mechanism is most likely to be relevant to attacks occurring after the onset of menstruation, particularly in association with menorrhagia and/or dysmenorrhoea.

Figure 13
Oestrogen withdrawal in 'menstrual' migraine. Source: Somerville (1972).

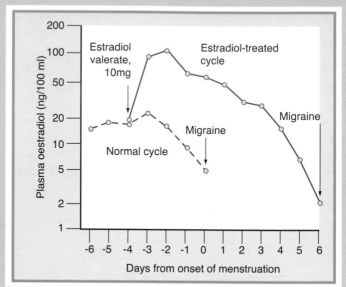

Figure 14
Progesterone in 'menstrual' migraine. Source: Somerville (1971).

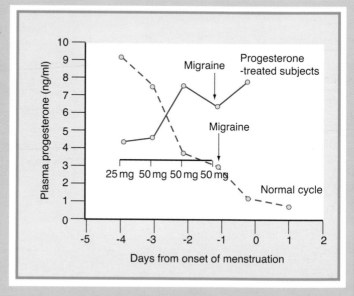

Management of suspected 'menstrual' migraine

First consultation

Once the diagnosis of migraine has been established, management strategies should include acute therapies, advice on non-hormonal trigger factors, and the provision of diary cards (Figure 15).

Attack therapy

Effective attack therapy may be all that is required if attacks are only occurring once a month. Standard acute treatments are recommended. However, there is evidence that menstrual attacks are less responsive to acute treatment than non-menstrual attacks (Figure 16).

Prophylaxis

Every effort should be made to identify and eliminate non-hormonal triggers where possible as this can reduce the likelihood of hormonal events triggering migraine (see the chapter: 'Who gets migraine and why?').

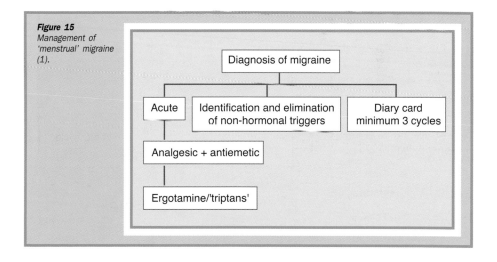

Figure 15
Management of 'menstrual' migraine (1).

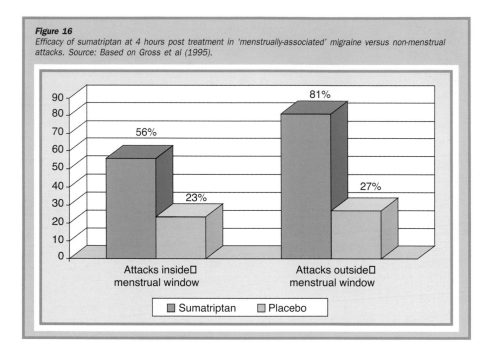

Figure 16
Efficacy of sumatriptan at 4 hours post treatment in 'menstrually-associated' migraine versus non-menstrual attacks. Source: Based on Gross et al (1995).

Diary cards

The most important aspect of management is to establish a true link between migraine and menstruation. Simple diary cards (Figures 17 and 18), kept for a minimum of three menstrual cycles, can be used to confirm or refute the association.

Subsequent consultation

By the time the diary cards are reviewed at follow-up, a percentage of patients will have their attacks under control, with no need for further intervention. Another group will have attacks throughout the cycle, which are not obviously related to menstruation. These women may benefit from standard prophylactic therapy, if considered necessary (Figure 19).

Only a small percentage of women will have 'menstrual' migraine requiring specific prophylaxis. Depending on

Figure 17
Diary card: no relation between migraine and irregular menstruation.

Figure 18
Diary card: 'menstrual' migraine and regular menstruation.

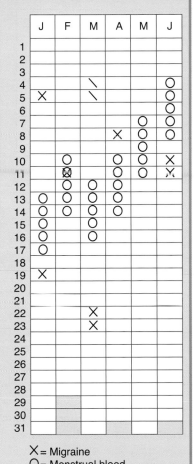

X = Migraine
O = Menstrual bleed
\ = Non-migraine headache

X = Migraine
O = Menstrual bleed
\ = Non-migraine headache

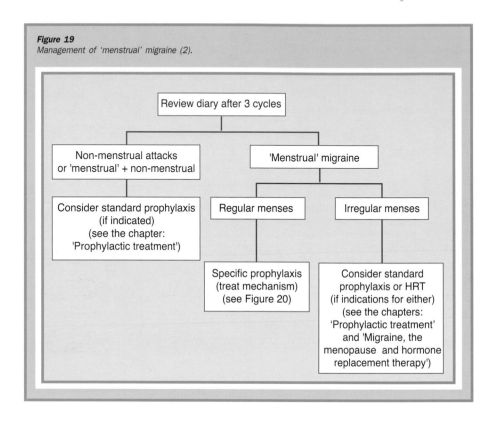

Figure 19
Management of 'menstrual' migraine (2).

each woman's wishes, the regularity of the menstrual cycle, timing of attacks in relation to bleeding, presence of dysmenorrhoea or menorrhagia, presence of menopausal symptoms, or need for contraception, several options can be tried, both non-hormonal and hormonal. Prophylaxis should be tried for a minimum of three cycles, increasing to maximum dose, before being deemed ineffective. No drug is universally effective or tolerated; therefore, each regimen should be tailored to the individual patient.

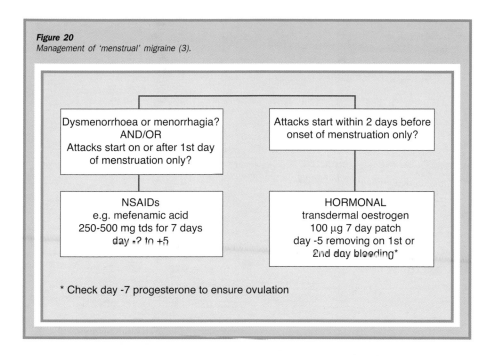

Figure 20
Management of 'menstrual' migraine (3).

Dysmenorrhoea or menorrhagia?
AND/OR
Attacks start on or after 1st day
of menstruation only?

Attacks start within 2 days before
onset of menstruation only?

NSAIDs
e.g. mefenamic acid
250-500 mg tds for 7 days
day -2 to +5

HORMONAL
transdermal oestrogen
100 μg 7 day patch
day -5 removing on 1st or
2nd day bleeding*

* Check day -7 progesterone to ensure ovulation

Specific prophylaxis for 'menstrual' migraine

If specific prophylaxis is indicated, the following methods can be tried (Figure 20). Note that none of the drugs and hormones recommended are licensed for management of menstrual migraine. Each regimen should be used for three cycles before being deemed ineffective. The alternative method can then be tried. If neither works, consider continuous hormonal methods discussed below or standard prophylaxis.

Non-steroidal anti-inflammatory drugs (NSAIDs)

NSAIDs are effective prostaglandin inhibitors. They should be tried as first-line agents for migraine attacks that start on the first to third day of bleeding. Side-effects include gastrointestinal disturbance. Contraindications include peptic ulcers and aspirin-induced allergy. Interactions include anticoagulants and antihypertensive agents.

Mefenamic acid is probably the drug of choice, 500 mg three to four times daily. This should be started either 2–3 days before the expected onset of menstruation, or started on the first day of bleeding. This should be taken for 2–3 days when bleeding is heavy, but can be used for the duration of menstrual bleeding. It is particularly helpful in reducing associated menorrhagia and/or dysmenorrhoea.

Some studies have suggested naproxen 550 mg once or twice daily from 7 days before menstruation for a total of 14 days.

Alternatively, fenoprofen 600 mg can be taken twice daily from 3 days before the onset of menstruation until the last day of bleeding.

Oestrogen supplements

If menstruation is irregular and associated with menopausal symptoms, HRT can be considered, as discussed in a later section.

If menstruation is regular and predictable, perimenstrual oestrogen supplements can be used to prevent the natural oestrogen drop in the late luteal phase of the menstrual cycle. Although this regimen uses treatments normally given for HRT, it is important to note that for 'menstrual' migraine, hormones are given as supplements. Provided the woman is ovulating regularly, no additional progestogens are necessary. This is because she will be producing adequate amounts of her own natural progesterone to counter the effects of unopposed oestrogen, which could otherwise lead to endometrial proliferation and hyperplasia. Ovulation can be confirmed, if necessary, with blood levels of progesterone taken 7 days before expected menstruation, i.e. day 21 of a 28-day cycle. The level should be greater than 30 nmol per litre. Side-effects due to excess oestrogen include breast tenderness, fluid retention, nausea, and leg cramps.

Transdermal oestrogen 100 µg can be used from approximately 3 days before expected menstruation for about 7 days, i.e. two twice-weekly patches or one 7-day patch. If this regimen is effective but side-effects are a problem, a 50 μg dose should be tried for the next cycle.

Alternatively, oestradiol gel 1.5 mg in 2.5 g gel can be applied daily from 3 days before expected menstruation for 7 days. This regimen may be more effective than transdermal patches as the gel produces higher, more stable, levels of oestrogen. However, it is less convenient for most women than patches.

Oestrogen supplements should not be used by women who are at risk of pregnancy, have undiagnosed vaginal bleeding, or oestrogen-dependent tumours.

Triptans

One open study used prophylactic oral sumatriptan 25mg three times daily given perimenstrually for 5 days to 20 women who reported a predictable association between migraine and menstruation and who had shown a past response to sumatriptan. In 126 sumatriptan-treated cycles, headache was absent in 52.4 per cent of cycles (Figure 21).

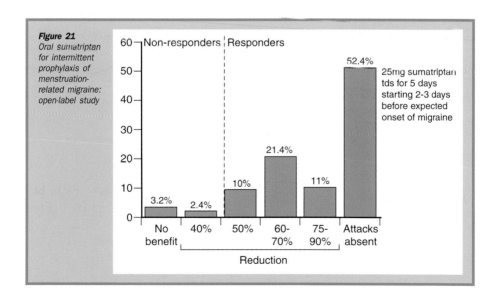

Figure 21
Oral sumatriptan for intermittent prophylaxis of menstruation-related migraine: open-label study

A more recent double-blind placebo controlled study of prophylactic naratriptan 1mg or 2.5 mg given perimenstrually for 5 days revealed that headache was absent in 23 per cent of cycles in women using the 1mg dose compared to a placebo response of 8 per cent (Figure 22). Interestingly, naratriptan 2.5 mg was no more effective than placebo.

Despite these good results, prophylactic use of triptans is not recommended until results of double-blind placebo-controlled trials confirm these findings.

Continuous hormonal strategies

If cycles are irregular, or the above strategies are ineffective despite a convincing hormonal link, the following methods can be considered. Several of these regimens are contraceptive.

Combined oral contraception (COC) inhibits ovulation, producing fairly stable oestrogen levels when taken, and can improve migraine in some women. Standard COC prescribing recommendations should be followed. Recommendations relating to use of

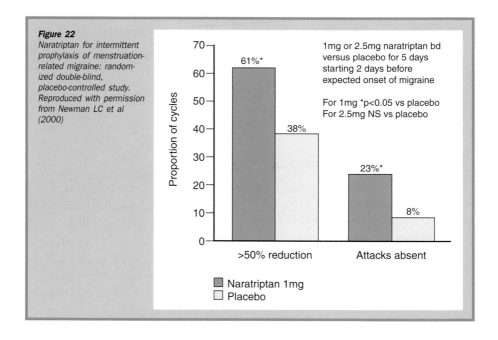

Figure 22
Naratriptan for intermittent prophylaxis of menstruation-related migraine: randomized double-blind, placebo-controlled study. Reproduced with permission from Newman LC et al (2000)

1mg or 2.5mg naratriptan bd versus placebo for 5 days starting 2 days before expected onset of migraine

For 1mg *p<0.05 vs placebo
For 2.5mg NS vs placebo

COCs in women with migraine are discussed in the chapter 'Migraine and contraception'.

Levonorgestrel (Mirena®) Intra-uterine System (IUS) is licensed for contraception but is also highly effective at reducing menstrual bleeding and associated pain. It can be considered for migraine related to dysmenorrhoea and/or menorrhagia. It is not effective for women who are sensitive to oestrogen withdrawal as a migraine trigger, as the majority of women still ovulate with the system in situ. Systemic effects are usually minor but erratic bleeding and spotting are common in the early months of use. Most women are amenorrhoeic within 1 year.

Injectable depot progestogens inhibit ovulation, similar to the mode of action of COCs. Although irregular bleeding can occur in early months of treatment, this method has the advantage that in most cases menstruation ceases. By inhibiting the normal menstrual cycle, hormonal triggers are removed. A few women appear to be sensitive to progestogens, developing premenstrual-type symptoms, although this is less likely with progesterone derivatives such as medroxyprogesterone acetate than with testosterone derivatives such as norethisterone.

Oral progestogen-only contraception has little place in the management of 'menstrual' migraine. It has no effect on potential mechanisms for 'menstrual' migraine, it does not inhibit ovulation, and is associated with a disrupted menstrual cycle.

Gonadotrophin-releasing hormones have been tried but side-effects of oestrogen deficiency (e.g. hot flushes), restrict their use. They are also associated with a marked reduction in bone density and should not usually be used regularly for longer than 6 months without regular monitoring and bone densitometry. Add-back continuous combined oestrogen and progestogen can be given to counter these difficulties. Given these limitations, in addition to increased cost, such treatment is best instigated in specialist departments.

Hysterectomy has no place in the management of migraine alone. Studies show that migraine is more likely to deteriorate after surgical menopause with bilateral oophorectomy. Even if an oophorectomy is not performed, hysterectomy often precipitates an early menopause. However, if other medical problems require surgical menopause, the effects may be lessened by subsequent oestrogen replacement therapy.

Key points

- The link between migraine and menstruation should be established using diary cards before considering hormonal therapy.
- Effective attack therapy alone may be sufficient for monthly attacks.
- Consider standard prophylaxis if attacks occur several times through the cycle.
- The choice of prophylaxis depends on the regularity of the menstrual cycle, the timing of attacks in relation to bleeding, the presence of dysmenorrhoea or menorrhagia, the presence of menopausal symptoms, and the need for contraception.
- There is no place for hysterectomy in the routine management of 'menstrual' migraine.

Migraine and the premenstrual syndrome

8

Distinct from attacks clustering around the first day of menstrual bleeding, migraine and other headaches are also associated with the premenstrual syndrome (also known as premenstrual dysphoric disorder) (Figure 23). Migraine occurs in the luteal phase of the menstrual cycle, following ovulation, and is associated with other premenstrual symptoms such as abdominal distension, breast tenderness, depression, and irritability.

Diagnosis

The diagnosis of premenstrual syndrome must be confirmed with diary cards, kept for at least three cycles. These should show a pattern of symptoms only during the second half of the menstrual cycle, relieved by menstruation.

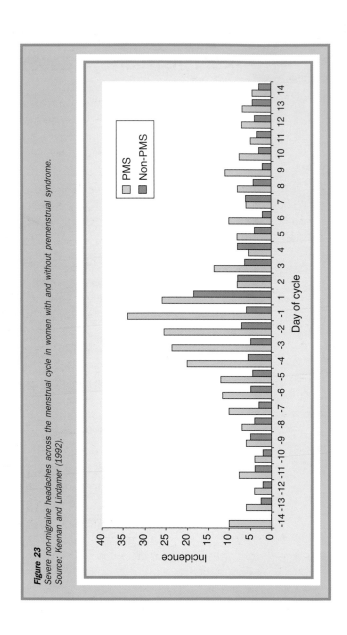

Figure 23
Severe non-migraine headaches across the menstrual cycle in women with and without premenstrual syndrome.
Source: Keenan and Lindamer (1992).

Management

Acute migraine treatment should be provided and optimized while treatment of premenstrual syndrome is tried.

Non-drug

The psychological 'cue' of menstruation is important as studies have shown improvement in premenstrual syndrome in women who have had an hysterectomy with conservation of the ovaries, i.e. the ovarian cycle has continued without bleeding as evidence. Therefore, initial management should be conservative, with many women responding to simple non-drug strategies including relaxation, psychotherapy, acupuncture, and yoga. General health advice to take regular exercise and eat frequent carbohydrate snacks may help–there is evidence that some women experience impaired glucose tolerance curve at this stage of the menstrual cycle.

Non-hormonal drugs

Many drugs have been used for the treatment of premenstrual symptoms but few are effective. This is particularly the case for pyridoxine (vitamin B6) which, although widely advocated, has limited value for this condition. There has been concern about high-dose vitamin B6 and over-the-counter doses are restricted. Doses over 500 mg per day have been associated with peripheral neuropathy. Indigestion and gastritis have also been reported in doses over 100 mg daily. Women wishing to try vitamin B6 are recommended to start with 50 mg once or twice daily and should not exceed 200 mg daily. This should be started about 10–14 days before the expected onset of menses but may be taken continuously if cycles are irregular.

Similarly, there is little evidence to confirm subjective reports of the efficacy of diuretics or progestogens in the management of premenstrual syndrome. Natural progesterone has been recommended but sedation is a common side-effect.

Magnesium pyrrolidone carboxylic acid 360 mg daily from mid-cycle to onset of menstruation has been effective for migraine and premenstrual symptoms but is not easily available in the UK. However, some women report that vitamin supplements containing magnesium are effective.

Oil of evening primrose, which contains gamolenic acid, a precursor of prostaglandins, is effective for cyclical mastalgia in doses of 120–160 mg twice daily and may reduce frequency of migraine.

St John's wort is used for depression, with few associated side-effects. It could be tried for premenstrual syndrome with associated depression in a dose of 300 mg solid extract three times daily.

SSRIs e.g. fluoxetine (20 mg daily), have shown encouraging results, particularly if depression coexists. If triptans are prescribed concomitantly, appropriate observation of the patient is advised.

Bromocriptine up to 7.5 mg daily in divided doses has been used for premenstrual and menstrual migraine but side-effects are a limiting factor.

Hormonal treatments

Hormonal treatments for premenstrual symptoms are used to alter or eliminate the natural ovarian cycle. These are similar to treatments used for confirmed 'menstrual' migraine and are discussed in more detail in that section. If menstruation is regular, oestrogen supplements can be given in a dose of 25–100 µg every 3–4 days. This should be started 7–10 days before the expected onset of menstruation and stopped shortly after the onset of bleeding.

Hormonal treatments that eliminate the ovarian cycle have been tried but there are few clinical data available on efficacy. These include injectable depot progestogens and COCs. Gonadotrophin-releasing hormone agonists are the most reliable means to suppress ovarian activity, inducing a 'reversible' menopause. In extreme cases, total abdominal hysterectomy with bilateral oophorectomy has been performed, following response to gonadotrophin-releasing hormone agonists. Subsequent oestrogen replacement should be prescribed.

Key points

- Migraine and headaches can occur as part of the premenstrual syndrome.
- Onset of symptoms subsequent to ovulation and relieved with menstruation should be confirmed using diary cards.
- Acute migraine treatment may be sufficient to control attacks.
- Conservative methods are the mainstay of management of premenstrual syndrome.
- Hormonal treatments should only be considered for severe symptoms.

Migraine and contraception

9

In the same way that a woman's own hormones affect migraine, so does hormonal contraception–but not always for the worse.

Oral contraception

There are two, quite differing, oral contraceptives. It is important to establish which method a woman is using as each has different implications for migraine.

Combined oral contraceptives (COCs) (Figure 24)

Headache is a frequent side-effect during the early months of COC use but usually resolves with continued use. With regard to migraine, COCs have a varying effect:

· No change	· More severe/frequent migraine
· Improvement in migraine	· Onset of migraine *de novo*
· Migraine in the pill-free interval	· Onset of aura *de novo*

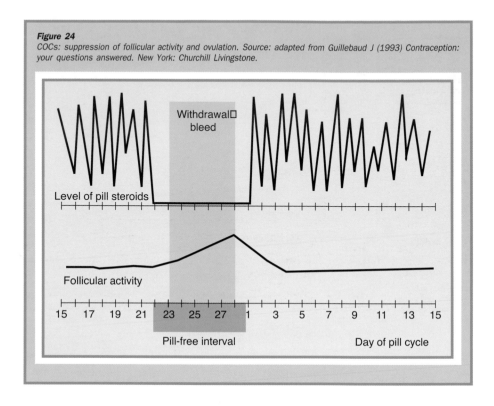

Figure 24
COCs: suppression of follicular activity and ovulation. Source: adapted from Guillebaud J (1993) Contraception: your questions answered. New York: Churchill Livingstone.

Some women report improvement but others note a worsening in frequency or severity of migraine with a tendency for attacks to occur during the pill-free interval.

For the majority of women COCs are a highly effective and safe method of contraception, with added health benefits such as protection against endometrial and ovarian cancer and certain sexually transmitted diseases. Results of recent studies suggest that migraine is associated with an increased risk of stroke, further increased by COCs, although the absolute risk remains very low in young women (Figure 25 and Table 9). These risks are further increased if the woman has other risk factors, particularly smoking.

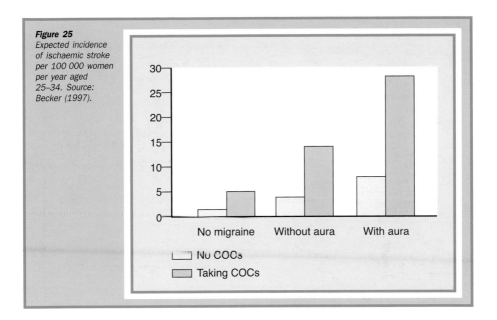

Figure 25
Expected incidence of ischaemic stroke per 100 000 women per year aged 25–34. Source: Becker (1997).

Prescribing COCs to women with migraine

In the UK, recommendations have been made to ensure safe prescribing of COCs by identifying women at risk of arterial thrombosis and offering alternative contraception (Figure 26). Owing to the increasing choice of methods available, there should be no loss of contraceptive efficacy (Table 10).

The terms 'focal' and 'simple' migraine used in family planning circles are equivalent to 'migraine with aura' and 'migraine without aura', respectively.

Reducing COC risks:

> • Some risks factors can be avoided:
>   – Smoking cessation
>   – Weight loss
>   – Control of hypertension and diabetes
> • Altnerative methods available, some of which are more effective than COCs:
>   – injectable progestogens, implants, levonorgestrel intrauterine system, intrauterine device

Table 9
Odds Ratios (OR) for ischaemic stroke.

	OR migraine (95%CI) [no. cases/ controls]	ethinyl-oestradiol (mcg)	OR COC use (95%CI) [no. cases/ controls]	OR COC use + migraine¶ (95%CI) [no. cases/ controls]
CGSS (1975)	2.0 RR* (1.2–3.3)[30/113]	≥50	4.9 RR (2.9–8.3)[41/38]	5.9 RR (2.9–12.2)[18/15]
Tzourio et al (1995)	3.5 (1.8–6.4)[43/52] with or without aura** 3.0 (1.5–5.8)[33/42] without aura** 6.2 (2.1–18.0)[10/10] with aura**	All doses 50 30–40 20	3.1 (1.2–8.2) 4.8 2.7 1.7	13.9 (5.5–35.1) – – –
Lidegaard (1993 and 1995)	2.8 with or without aura***	All doses 50 30–40	– 2.9(1.6–5.4) 1.8(1.1–2.9)	5 – –
Carolei et al (1996)	1.3 with or without aura** (0.7–2.4) 3.7(1.5–9.0) if <35yrs 8.6(1–75) with aura 1.0(0.5–2.0) without aura	All doses	1.3(0.6–2.6)	no data
WHO Collabora-tive study (1996)	no data	All doses (Europe) ≥50 <50	2.24(1.31–3.82) [52/87] 5.3(2.56–11.0) [32/35] 1.53(0.71–3.31) [20/52]	no data
Chang et al (1999)	2.97(0.66–13.5)[7/9] without aura** 3.81(1.26–11.5)[19/17] with aura**	All doses ≥50 <50	2.76(1.01–7.55) [19/42] 7.95(1.94–32.6) [9/14] 1.19(0.33–4.29) [10/28]	16.9(2.72–106) [10/3] Cannot be calculated 6.59(0.79 to 54.8) [4/3]

95%CI = 95 per cent confidence intervals; RR = relative risk; *diagnosis based on presence of two or more of the following symptoms: unilateral headache, throbbing quality, visual scintillation, vomiting, and other symptoms (study predates IHS criteria); **diagnosis made using IHS criteria; ***self-reported diagnosis; attack frequency > 1 per month; ¶ data not differentiated for ethinyloestradiol dose.

Figure 26
Recommendations for use of COCs in women with migraine. Source: MacGregor, Guillebaud (1998).

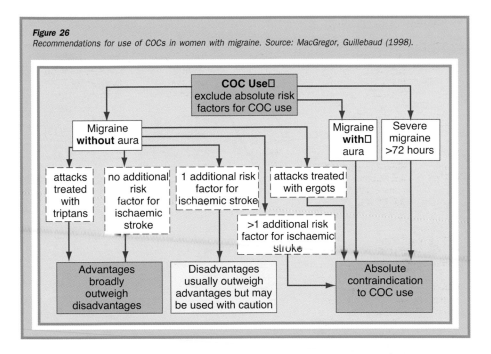

Table 10
Failure rates of contraception per 100 woman – years.

Contraceptive method	Failure rate
COC	0.2–3
POP	1–4
Levonorgestrel IUS	0–0.2
Injectable DMPA	0–1
Implant	0–1
IUD (Cu-T380)	0.3–0.5
Sterilization	
Male	0–0.2
Female	0–1
No method, young women	80–90

Source: Based on Guillebaud (2000).

Advantages of COCs outweigh disadvantages:

> • *Migraine without aura in a woman with no additional risk factors for stroke*, provided there is no marked increase in migraine frequency or severity associated with COC use.
> • *Use of triptans for acute treatment*, provided there are no other contraindications to COC or triptan use as specified in the data sheets.

Use COCs with caution:

> *Migraine without aura in a woman who has a history of one additional relative risk factor for stroke*, since multiple factors increase the risk of ischaemic stroke, particularly smoking. If additional risk factors are noted, COCs should be discontinued (Tables 11 and 12).

Contraindications to COC use

These apply to pre-existing migraine and conditions that develop during COC use:

> • *Migraine with aura* because the limited data available suggest that the risk of ischaemic stroke associated with migraine with aura in a COC user is greater than the risk associated with pregnancy. Consequently, the Faculty of Family Planning in the UK consider the presence of focal neurological symptoms to be a contraindication to COC use. This risk is associated with synthetic oestrogen; therefore progestogen-only and non-hormonal methods can be offered. Women with a distant past history of migraine with aura, such as during childhood, may be offered a trial of COCs but these should be discontinued immediately if focal neurological symptoms occur. Differences between migraine aura and ischaemic symptoms are discussed in the chapters 'What is migraine?' and 'Clinical diagnosis'.
> • *Migraine without aura in a woman who has a history of two or more additional risk factors for stroke.*
> • *Severe migraine/'status migrainosus'* defined as attacks of migraine which are unusually severe and last longer than 72 hours, despite treatment. In these situations it may be difficult to distinguish clearly between severe migraine and organic cerebral ischaemia. If medication misuse is excluded or if appropriate investigations (if indicated) exclude underlying pathology, a further trial of COCs may be considered.
> • *Concurrent use of ergots*, since this class of drugs has widespread vasoconstrictor effects which, coupled with the prothrombotic effect of COCs, increase the risk of thrombotic stroke.

Table 11
Relative contraindications to the use of COCs.

Risk factor	Relative contraindication
Family history of arterial/venous disease (in a first-degree relative aged ≤ 45 years)	Normal lipid and/or haemostatic profile or first attack in relative aged > 45
Diabetes mellitus	No 'opathies'
Hypertension	BP ≤ 160/95
Smoking	5–40/day
Age	Non-smokers aged 35–50
Weight	BMI ≥ 30
Migraine	• Treatment with triptan • Without aura if no risk factor • (Caution if one risk factor)

Note: More than one contraindication = absolute contraindication.
Source: Based on Guillebaud (1998).

Table 12
Absolute contraindications to the use of COCs.

Risk factor	Absolute contraindication
Family history of arterial/venous disease (in a first-degree relative aged ≤ 45 years)	• Abnormal lipid and/or haemostatic profile • Tests not available
Diabetes mellitus	'Opathies' present
Hypertension	BP > 160/95 on repeat testing
Smoking	40+ cigarettes/day
Age	Non-smokers aged > 50
Weight	BMI > 39
Migraine	• Aura • 'Status migrainosus' • Treatment with ergotamine • Without aura if more than one additional risk factor

Source: Based on Guillebaud (1998).

Migraine in the pill-free week

Migraine occurring exclusively in the pill-free week is probably triggered by falling levels of ethinyloestradiol. Such attacks are typically migraine without aura and usually commence a couple of days after the last pill is taken. If acute treatment is inadequate to control symptoms, hormonal prophylaxis may be considered. Although there are no data from clinical trials to support the following suggestions, they are widely used in clinical practice. The tricycle regimen of three consecutive pill packets followed by a pill-free interval means that the woman has only 5 such migraines a year instead of 13. COCs may be taken continuously, without a break, although breakthrough bleeding may occur. However, there are advantages to regular pill-free intervals as these provide a break from the metabolic effects of COCs. Therefore natural oestrogen supplements such as 100 µg transdermal patches, 1.5 mg percutaneous gel, or 2 mg oral oestradiol valerate daily during the pill-free interval provide some protection against oestrogen withdrawal using natural oestrogen, while enabling a progestogen withdrawal bleed to occur.

Emergency contraception

The current recommendations in the UK state that combined hormonal postcoital contraception (PC4®) can be given provided a woman with a history of migraine with aura is not experiencing migraine at the time of treatment. This situation rarely occurs in practice but alternative methods such as levonorgestrel-only oral postcoital contraception (*note*: not the levonorgestrel intrauterine system) or a copper intrauterine device may be considered (Table 13).

Which COC for a migraineur?

Risk of ischaemic stroke is directly proportional to the dose of ethinyloestradiol; therefore the lowest acceptable dose should be given in line with current prescribing recommendations. With regard to progestogens, limited data suggest that migraine in the pill-free interval is most notable in women taking combined contraceptives that contain a relatively high proportion of progestogen. In these situations, an oestrogen-dominant pill may be considered.

Table 13
Emergency contraception.

Ethinyloestradiol (PC4):	contraindicated during an attack of migraine *only* if history of migraine with aura
Alternatives:	– progestogen-only
	– copper IUD (not IUS)

Note: UK recommendation only, WHO do not contraindicate migraine with aura

Progestogen-only pill (POP)

Unlike combined oral contraceptives which inhibit ovulation, many women taking the progestogen-only pill continue to ovulate but with erratic cycles. This can lead to menstrual irregularity which, together with headache, are common reasons for discontinuation of this method.

Injectables

Depot medroxyprogesterone acetate (DMPA) is the most commonly used injectable and is administered at 3-monthly intervals. Side-effects are common in early months of use, particularly menstrual irregularities. However, amenorrhoea is typical within one year of use and is often associated with improvement in migraine as ovulation is inhibited.

DMPA has the advantage of lower contraceptive failure rates than COCs but return to normal fertility takes an average of 6 months after the final dose.

Implants

Although this method has high contraceptive efficacy and is rapidly reversible, bleeding problems and headaches are common reasons for dissatisfaction with this method. Its use is not recommended in women with migraine without careful counselling of the possible effects on headache.

Intrauterine contraception

Two methods of intrauterine contraception are currently available which work by quite separate mechanisms.

Levonorgestrel-releasing intrauterine system (LNG-IUS)

The presence of a slow-releasing rod of levonorgestrel within the womb reduces menstrual bleeding such that many women are amenorrhoeic within one year of insertion. Despite amenorrhoea, most women continue to have normal ovarian cycles so oestrogen withdrawal may still occur as a migraine trigger. Headache and migraine are common in association with early menstrual disturbance but improve as bleeding settles.

Copper intrauterine devices

The standard copper intrauterine devices remain highly effective non-hormonal methods of contraception. The newer models such as the copper Gyne-T380® are more effective than COCs. However, they can cause increased and prolonged menstrual bleeding which may be associated with migraine.

Other non-hormonal methods

Sterilization, condoms, caps (diaphragms), and natural family planning methods have little effect on the normal hormonal cycle and therefore their use is not associated with any change in the pattern of migraine.

Key points

- COCs are safe for women with migraine without aura unless multiple risk factors for ischaemic stroke are present.
- COCs are contraindicated for women with migraine with aura.
- Progestogen-only and non-hormonal methods of contraception are not associated with an increased risk of ischaemic stroke.
- Some progestogen-only and non-hormonal methods are more effective contraceptives than the combined pill.

Migraine and pregnancy

10

Studies suggest that between 60 and 70% of migraineurs experience an improvement in their migraine during pregnancy, particularly during the second and third trimesters. The mechanism is often considered to be the more stable levels of oestrogen during pregnancy. However, it is unlikely that the true mechanism is so simple as there are many physical, biochemical, and emotional changes in pregnancy which could account for improvement, including increased production of endorphins, muscle relaxation, and altered glucose tolerance.

Migraine without aura

Women who have attacks of migraine without aura before becoming pregnant, particularly if they have noticed a link between migraine and menstruation, are most likely to notice a respite from migraine during pregnancy. This typically continues during lactation until the return of menses, although migraine associated with the sudden drop in oestrogen immediately post-partum is not uncommon. But not every woman with migraine without aura improves during pregnancy–around 16% continue to have attacks throughout.

Migraine with aura

In contrast to migraine without aura, women who have pre-existing migraine with aura are more likely to continue to have attacks during pregnancy. Also, if migraine starts for the first time during pregnancy, it is likely to be with aura.

Differential diagnosis

Other disorders, such as thrombocy-topenia, cerebral venous sinus throm-bosis, or imminent eclampsia, may present with symptoms not dissimilar from migraine. To avoid incorrect diagnosis, a careful history and exami-nation are mandatory, particularly if symptoms change or the first attack starts during pregnancy. As in the non-pregnant state, several headaches can coexist, in which case each headache should be diagnosed and treated separately.

Reassurance

There is no evidence that migraine, either with or without aura, has any effect on the outcome of pregnancy. Of more potential concern are women who develop aura for the first time during pregnancy. Provided the diagnosis of migraine is confirmed and other conditions are ruled out, case studies show that typical aura does not appear to be associated with sinister sequelae.

Once the diagnosis of migraine has been confirmed, the first step in management is to reassure the patient that migraine does not pose any threat to the baby. This is particularly impor-tant for women with attacks of migraine with aura who may fear a stroke or other condition posing a threat to the pregnancy.

Non-drug management

Many pregnant women favour non-drug methods of management while they are pregnant, particularly once they are aware that migraine is likely to improve. Early pregnancy symptoms can aggravate migraine. Pregnancy sickness, particularly if severe, can reduce food and fluid intake resulting in low blood sugar and dehydration. Simple advice to eat small, frequent carbohydrate snacks and drink plenty of fluids may help both problems. Adequate rest is necessary to counter overtiredness, particularly in the first and last trimesters. Other preventative measures that can safely be tried include acupuncture, biofeedback, yoga, massage, and relaxation techniques.

Herbal remedies

Many people equate 'natural' with 'safe' and are not aware that medicinal herbs can be powerful drugs. Some drugs used in migraine, such as feverfew, have the potential to cause miscarriage. For these reasons, patients should be warned to avoid herbal medicines unless recommended by a qualified practitioner.

Drug management

Few drugs have been tested for safety in pregnancy and during breast-feeding because of the obvious ethical limitations of undertaking clinical trials. This lack of data means that manufacturers do not generally recommend the use of any drug in pregnancy. Therefore, use of most drugs in pregnancy is unlicensed.

To avoid the potential for drug-related effects on pregnancy, it is important to minimize drug exposure whenever conception is possible. Drugs should only be considered if the potential benefits to the woman and fetus outweigh the potential risks. Many drugs and other teratogens exert their greatest effects on the fetus in the first trimester, often before the woman knows she is pregnant. If possible, prophylactic medication should be discontinued and strategies for the management of acute attacks discussed with any woman who is planning pregnancy or who is at high risk of unplanned pregnancy. As few drugs as possible should be used that have the least potential to cause damage, and in the lowest effective dose.

If a drug is taken, at any stage of pregnancy, it is essential the woman is provided with sufficient information about any known risks, in order that she can make her own decision about its use. This should be documented in her notes. Women who have taken their usual migraine treatment will be concerned about the effects of these and other drugs on the pregnancy and should be reassured where possible.

Migraine drugs in pregnancy

These recommendations are based on a literature review (Table 14). Manufacturers' usual advice is to avoid drug use during pregnancy. In the UK, further advice is available from local drug information centres, the National Drug Information Service and from the National Teratology Information Service (see 'Useful Information', p. 79).

Analgesics

Aspirin Clinical and epidemiological data from large numbers of women who have taken analgesic doses of aspirin during pregnancy provide evidence of its safety in the first and second trimesters of pregnancy. It should be used with caution near term as its effect on platelet function increases the risk of prolonged labour, post-partum haemorrhage, and neonatal bleeding. In common with all prostaglandin synthetase inhibitors, aspirin may cause premature closure of the fetal ductus arteriosus.

Codeine Respiratory malformation in neonates may be associated with codeine exposure during pregnancy. However, occasional use at doses found in combined analgesics is unlikely to cause harm.

Ibuprofen Animal studies with ibuprofen have not shown any treatment-related abnormalities and the drug has been safely given during pregnancy at doses not exceeding 600 mg daily for the management of rheumatoid arthritis. Other effects are similar to those of aspirin.

NSAIDs There are insufficient data to support the use of most NSAIDs in pregnant women.

Paracetamol Paracetamol is the mild analgesic of choice in pregnancy provided it is not taken in combination with methionine, a drug used to prevent paracetamol toxicity.

Antiemetics

Buclizine is an antihistamine combined with paracetamol and codeine in an over-the-counter migraine treatment. Although it has been in wide use for many years without apparent adverse effects, controlled data are limited.

Cyclizine is also widely available without prescription alone or in combination with analgesics for the

Table 14
Common migraine drugs: use during pregnancy and lactation.

	First Trimester	Second Trimester	Third Trimester	Lactation
Aspirin	(√)	(√)	avoid	avoid
Codeine	(√)	(√)	(√)	√
Ibuprofen	(√)	(√)	avoid	(√)
NSAIDs	ID	ID	avoid	(√)
Paracetamol	√	√	√	√
Buclizine	ID	ID	ID	ID
Cyclizine	ID	ID	ID	ID
Domperidone	(√)	(√)	(√)	√
Metoclopramide	(√)	(√)	(√)	avoid
Prochlorperazine	(√)	(√)	(√)	(√)
Ergotamine	C/I	C/I	C/I	C/I
Dihydroergotamine	C/I	C/I	C/I	C/I
Triptans	ID	ID	ID	ID*
Amitriptyline	avoid	(√)	avoid	avoid
Methysergide	C/I	C/I	C/I	C/I
Pizotifen	(√)	(√)	(√)	(√)
Propanolol	(√)	(√)	(√)	(√)
Valproate	C/I	C/I	C/I	C/I
Verapamil	C/I	(√)	(√)	√

ID = insufficient data; C/I = contraindicated; (√) = probably safe; √ = no evidence of risk.
* Rizatriptan data sheet recommends avoiding breast-feeding for 24 hours after treatment.
Source: Adapted from MacGregor (1994).

treatment of migraine but, again, controlled data are limited. It is a possible teratogen although this concern has not been substantiated in prospective controlled studies.

Variable embryotoxic effects have occurred in animal tests but a causal link with *domperidone* has not been confirmed. A study of 50 pregnant women treated over 20 days between the fourth and twelfth week of pregnancy showed no adverse outcome.

Metoclopramide has not shown any teratogenic effect in clinical experience or in animal studies.

Prochlorperazine has been widely used without ill-effect and animal studies have not shown any teratogenic effect.

Vasoconstrictors

Ergotamine is contraindicated in pregnancy as animal studies have shown that its use is associated with increased perinatal mortality and developmental anomalies, including cleft palate and limb defects. This is thought to be the result of ergotamine's potent vasoconstrictor action, impairing uteroplacental blood flow. It

is also an abortifacient so should only be given to women using effective contraception. Ergotamine should not be taken during breast-feeding as it inhibits lactation.

Dihydroergotamine is not a known teratogen but, with limited data available, its use in pregnancy and during breast-feeding is not recommended.

Few women have taken *triptans* during pregnancy but there has been no evidence of teratogenicity. However, with such limited exposure, the use of triptans cannot be recommended during pregnancy.

Prophylactics

Amitriptyline has been used for management of major depressive illness during pregnancy when the illness may affect the well-being of the mother. For migraine it is probably best avoided and should not be used during the first and last trimesters. A few cases of limb deformity have been reported but this finding has not been confirmed by the results of national surveys. Tachycardia, irritability, muscle spasms, and convulsions have occasionally been reported in the neonate.

Methysergide has uterogenic properties. Its use is contraindicated in pregnancy and it should only be given to women using effective contraception.

Pizotifen has not been associated with any reported embryotoxic or adverse effects during pregnancy although the data are limited.

Propranolol has not been established to be safe in pregnancy, but has been widely taken with no evidence of teratogenicity and is the only prophylactic that can be recommended. Even so, its use should be restricted to severe cases not responding to non-drug management. Propranolol has been associated with growth retardation, hypoglycaemia, hypocalcaemia, bradycardia, and respiratory depression. Since most women are given propranolol in pregnancy for the treatment of hypertension or eclampsia, it is difficult to know if the underlying condition, or the treatment, is the cause of these effects. Other beta-blockers have similar effects but data are even more limited.

Valproate is highly teratogenic. Its use is contraindicated in pregnancy and it should only be given to women using effective contraception. First-trimester use is associated with neural tube defects and a characteristic pattern of facial defects.

Verapamil has only had limited use in pregnancy. There are no reported teratogenic effects but it can potentially cause fetal bradycardia.

Migraine drugs during lactation

Analgesics

- *Aspirin*: is excreted in breast milk so breast-feeding mothers should avoid its use because of the theoretical risk of Reye's syndrome and impaired platelet function in susceptible infants although occasional use by the mother is unlikely to cause adverse effects.
- *Codeine*: occasional use of over-the-counter drugs containing codeine is unlikely to cause harm although large doses of codeine excreted in the breast milk can cause sedation and respiratory depression
- *Ibuprofen*: the concentration of ibuprofen in breast milk is very low and is therefore unlikely to affect the infant.
- *NSAIDs*: data are too limited to recommend the use of other NSAIDs for migraine during lactation.
- *Paracetamol*: is the mild analgesic of choice in breast-feeding women. However, the combination with methionine is contraindicated during lactation, as in pregnancy.

Antiemetics

- *Buclizine*: minimal levels pass into breast milk so it can be taken during breast-feeding.
- *Cyclizine*: there is no evidence to suggest that cyclizine cannot be used during lactation.
- *Domperidone*: minimal amounts are excreted into breast milk and domperidone is occasionally prescribed to improve postnatal lactation.
- *Metoclopramide*: although only small amounts are found in breast milk and are unlikely to produce adverse effects, its use should be avoided in favour of domperidone.
- *Prochlorperazine*: there is no evidence to suggest that prochlorperazine cannot be used during lactation.

Prophylactics

- *Amitriptyline*: is detectable in breast milk but the effects on the neonate are unknown.
- *Methysergide*: is contraindicated during lactation.
- *Pizotifen*: safety during breast-feeding is not established although concentrations of pizotifen measured in breast milk are not likely to affect the infant adversely.
- *Propranolol*: is not significantly excreted into breast milk and its use is not therefore absolutely contraindicated in breast-feeding women. However, attention should be paid to the infant in case of bradycardia and hypoglycaemia.
- *Valproate*: the concentration found in breast milk is very low so it can be used during lactation.
- *Verapamil*: there is no evidence of any risk associated with the use of verapamil during lactation.

Vasoconstrictors

- *Ergotamine*: should not be taken during breastfeeding as it inhibits lactation.
- *Dihydroergotamine*: data are too limited to make a recommendation.
- *Triptans*: data are too limited to recommend use of most triptans during lactation, although the data sheets suggest that infant exposure can be minimized by avoiding breast-feeding for 24 hours after treatment.

Prescribing for the pregnant woman

Although many of the drugs taken by unsuspecting pregnant women rarely cause harm, there is a difference between reassuring the pregnant woman that what she has taken is unlikely to have affected the pregnancy, and advising her what she should take for future attacks. For acute treatment, paracetamol is safe throughout pregnancy and lactation. Aspirin is also safe, but may cause bleeding problems if taken near term. Prochlorperazine has been used for pregnancy-related nausea for many years. Metoclopramide and domperidone are safe, but are probably best avoided during the first trimester. If frequent attacks occur during the first trimester, most women can be reassured that migraine improves during the second and third trimesters. For continuing frequent attacks, which warrant prophylaxis, propranolol has

best evidence of safety during pregnancy and lactation.

Key points

- Use of drugs in pregnancy is a balance of risks and benefits.
- Paracetamol is safe during pregnancy and lactation.
- Domperidone and prochlorperazine can be taken for nausea during pregnancy and lactation, but there is less evidence for the safety of domperidone.
- Propranolol is the drug of choice if prophylaxis is necessary during pregnancy and lactation.

Migraine, the menopause, and hormone replacement therapy

11

The perimenopause marks a time of exacerbation of migraine for many women. Menstruation becomes a more prominent trigger with regular monthly migraine attacks. The onset of irregular menses can make it harder for a woman to cope as migraine is no longer predictable. Further, there is often the additional problem of hot flushes, night sweats, and other menopausal symptoms.

For some women, effective attack therapy and an explanation about the probable cause of worsening migraine may be sufficient, as cessation of menses following the natural menopause usually marks a time of improvement.

Others, particularly women with severe migraine and menopausal symptoms or those with exacerbation of migraine following surgical menopause, may wish to consider HRT.

Management strategies for perimenopausal migraine

As with 'menstrual' migraine, diary cards are important to diagnosis and management (Figure 27). First, they can help to establish a link between menses, menopausal symptoms, and migraine. During the 3 months these are being completed, attack therapy can be recommended and non-hormonal triggers identified and managed.

If the diary cards do not suggest an hormonal link, or there are no menopausal symptoms but attacks are troublesome with inadequate response to acute treatments, standard prophy-laxis may be considered. If attacks linked to irregular menses or other menopausal symptoms are apparent, the woman may wish to try HRT, provided there are no contraindications to its use. These include undiagnosed vaginal bleeding, oestrogen-dependent cancers, and active aterial or venous disease.

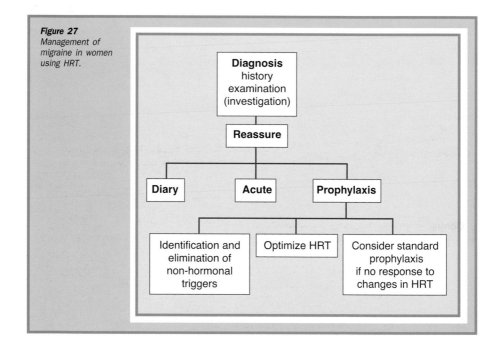

Figure 27
Management of migraine in women using HRT.

Hormone replacement therapy and migraine

It is a commonly held belief that HRT will aggravate migraine. This is certainly true if HRT is prescribed without consideration of the potential hormonal triggering mechanisms of migraine.

Oestrogen

Studies suggest that non-oral routes of delivery of oestrogen are more likely to improve migraine than oral oestrogens (Table 15). Oral oestrogens are associated with wide day-to-day variations in serum concentrations (Figure 28). These fluctuations could play a part in triggering migraine, particularly if coupled with a background of fluctuating endogenous oestrogens in perimenopausal women. Conversely, non-oral routes such as transdermal or percutaneous routes are associated with more stable oestrogen levels at physiological doses (Figure 29). Oestradiol implants are only recommended for use in hysterectomized women because of their long duration of effect on the endometrium. It is important to ensure that an adequate dose of oestrogen is given to

Table 15
Effects of oral and transdermal oestrogen replacement on migraine.

	% of users		
	Better	**Worse**	**No change**
Conjugated oral oestrogens + cyclical progestogen (Prempak C®) n=52	42	50	8
Transdermal oestradiol + cyclical progestogen (Prempak C®) n=26	69	23	8

Source: MacGregor (1999b).

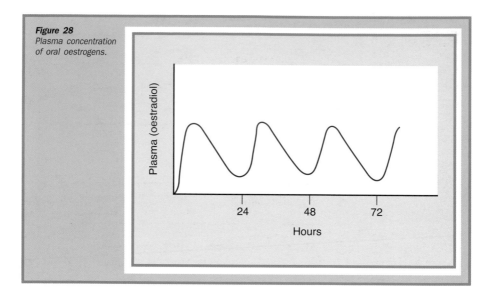

Figure 28
Plasma concentration of oral oestrogens.

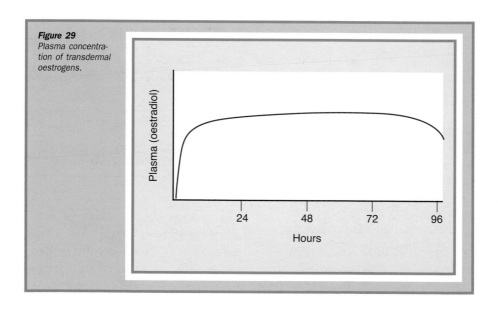

Figure 29
Plasma concentration of transdermal oestrogens.

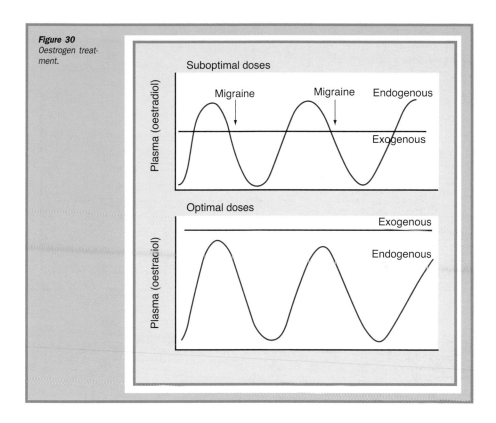

Figure 30
Oestrogen treatment.

limit endogenous oestrogen fluctuations (Figure 30). Tailoring treatment is a particular problem for perimenopausal women as too high a dose, coupled with surges of endogenous oestrogen, can result in symptoms of oestrogen excess including nausea, fluid retention, breast tenderness, and leg cramps. For optimal oestrogen replacement therapy:

- continuous oestrogen
- maintain stable levels
- maintain physiologic levels

High doses of oestrogen can occasionally trigger attacks of typical migraine aura. These symptoms usually resolve with a reduction in dose or change from an oral to a non-oral route.

Natural oestrogens are considered to reduce the risk of arterial thrombosis, although the benefits are no longer as certain as was initially thought. However, there is no evidence that physiological doses of natural oestrogens have the thrombotic potential of synthetic oestrogens at contraceptive doses. Consequently, there is no reason to contraindicate HRT in women with migraine with aura.

Progestogens

Additional progestogen is necessary to prevent endometrial cancer in unhysterectomized women using oestrogen replacement. However, side-effects are common, including premenstrual symptoms, headaches, and migraine (Figure 31). This is more of a problem with cyclical progestogens than with continuous combined regimens.

Figure 31
The diary card.

May	Day	Headache	Time started	How long it lasted	Did you feel sick?	Were you sick?	What tablets did you take?	Taken at what time?	HRT
1	Tue								
2	Wed								PATCH 4
3	Thu	Mild	8am	10am	No	No			
4	Fri								
5	Sat								
6	Sun								PATCH 5/ 1st pill
7	Mon								pill
8	Tue								pill
9	Wed								PATCH 6/ pill
10	Thu	Mild	8pm	bedtime	No				pill
11	Fri	Severe	4am	all day	Yes	Yes	Domperidone (1) Aspirin (3)	} 10am & 3pm	pill
12	Sat	Moderate	–	all day	Yes	No	Same as above	8am	pill
13	Sun								PATCH 7/ pill
14	Mon								pill

However, the latter is only indicated for postmenopausal women. Changing the type of progestogen can resolve the problem, as side-effects are fewer with progesterone derivatives such as medroxyprogesterone acetate and dydrogesterone than with testosterone derivatives such as norethisterone:

- progesterone derivative instead of testosterone derivative
- transdermal progestogens
- intravaginal progesterone
- levonorgestrel intra-uterine system
- 3-monthly, instead of monthly
- continuous combined in place of cyclical combined (postmenopause only)

Changing route from oral to transdermal progestogen can be effective. The course of cyclical progestogens could be reduced to only 7–10 days per month, although this increases the risk of endometrial hyperplasia. Alternatively, if natural periods are infrequent, progestogens could be limited to three-monthly cycles. Natural progesterone is also available as suppositories, vaginal gel, and, in some countries, as micronized tablets. The levonorgestrel intrauterine system (Mirena®) can provide the progestogen component with minimal systemic effects. Occasionally, progestogenic

side-effects are sufficient for a woman to choose to discontinue progestogens. In these cases, specialist care is appropriate because of the risk of endometrial hyperplasia and cancer.

Non-hormonal prophylaxis

Clonidine (50–75 µg twice daily) is licensed for menopausal hot flushes and migraine prophylaxis and may be useful for women not wishing, or unable, to take HRT. However, trial data to support its efficacy as a migraine prophylactic are limited. Side-effects include sedation, dry mouth, dizziness, and insomnia. As it is also antihypertensive, it should not be taken concomitantly with other antihypertensive agents.

When treatment fails

If migraine continues despite HRT being effective against hot flushes, and there is no pattern of migraine associated with progestogen cycles, it is unlikely that hormonal factors are an important migraine trigger. Sometimes migraine occurs only in association with the withdrawal bleed following progestogen therapy. Since oestrogen levels remain fairly stable with HRT, the most likely mechanism is prostaglandin release. Therefore, prostaglandin inhibitors could be prescribed during the withdrawal bleed, or the levonorgestrel intrauterine system used as adjunct progestogen therapy. If there is no hormonal pattern to frequent attacks and acute treatment alone is inadequate, standard migraine prophylaxis is indicated. Increased stresses, life changes, musculoskeletal problems, and depression are common in this age group and may be more important than hormonal triggers.

Key points

- Migraine is at peak prevalence in perimenopausal women.
- HRT can help migraine triggered by hormonal fluctuations.
- Non-oral oestrogens prescribed continuously in adequate doses are best for migraineurs.
- Progesterone derivatives, non-oral progestogens, or progesterone should be considered if migraine is associated with cyclical progestogens.

Useful information

Professional Organisations

International Headache Society (I.H.S.)
Membership includes subscription to *Cephalalgia*, an international headache journal.

For details of membership to IHS and information about national societies worldwide contact:
Rosemary Chilcott
Permanent Secretary
International Headache Society
'Oakwood'
9,Willowmead Drive
Prestbury
Cheshire
SK10 4BU, UK
Tel: +44 (0)1625 828663
Fax: +44 (0)1625 828494
Email: rosemary@ihs.u-net.com
Internet: www.i-h-s.org

Primary care

Migraine in Primary Care Advisors (MIPCA) Secretariat
Rebecca Salt
Surrey Headache Service
Merrow Park Surgery
Kingfisher Drive, Merrow
Guildford, Surrey, GU4 7EP
Tel: 01483 450755

Lay organizations

Worldwide:
World Headache Alliance
612 Thornwood Avenue
Burlington
Ontario, L7N 3B8
Tel +1 905 637 5254
Fax +1 905 333 8185
E-Mail WHAmail@AOL.com
Internet:
www.worldheadachealliance.org

United Kingdom:
Details on migraine clinics in the UK are available from both of the following organizations.

Migraine Action Association
Unit 6
Oakley Hay Lodge Business Park
Great Folds Road, Corby
NORTHANTS NN18 9AS
Tel: +44 (0)1536 461333; Fax: +44 (0)1536 461444
Internet: www.migraine.org.uk

The Migraine Trust
45 Great Ormond Street
LONDON WC1N 3HZ
Tel: +44 (0)20 7831 4818; Fax: +44 (0)20 7831 5174
Internet: www.migrainetrust.org

Clinic

The City of London Migraine Clinic
22 Charterhouse Square
LONDON EC1M 6DX
Tel: +44 (0)20 7251 3322; Fax: +44 (0)20 7490 2183
Internet: www.colmc.org.uk

National Teratology Information Service

Regional Drug and Therapeutics Centre
Wolfson Unit
Claremont Place
Newcastle-Upon-Tyne NE1 4LP
Tel: +44 (0)191 232 1525; Fax: +44 (0)191 261 5733

Sumatriptan and Naratriptan Pregnancy Registry

Patient Registries and Outreach Programs, PharmaResearch Corp.
Research Park - 1011 Ashes Drive
Wilmington, NC 28405
pregnancyregistry.gsk.com/naratriptan.html

International Headache Society diagnostic criteria

The following is adapted from Headache Classification Committee of the International Headache Society (1988).

Migraine without aura (common migraine)

A. At least five attacks fulfilling B–D.

B. Headache attacks, lasting 4–72 hours (untreated or unsuccessfully treated).

C. Headache has at least two of the following characteristics:

1) Unilateral location.
2) Pulsating quality.
3) Moderate or severe intensity (inhibits or prohibits daily activities).
4) Aggravation by walking stairs or similar routine activity.

D. During headache at least one of the following:

1) Nausea and/or vomiting.
2) Photophobia and phonophobia.

Migraine with aura (classical migraine)

A. At least two attacks fulfilling B.

B. At least three of the following four characteristics:

1) One or more fully reversible aura symptoms indicating focal cerebral cortical and/or brainstem dysfunction.
2) At least one aura symptom develops gradually over more than 4 minutes, or two or more symptoms occur in succession.
3) No aura symptom lasts more than 60 minutes. If more than one aura symptom is present, accepted duration is proportionally increased.
4) Headache follows aura with a free interval of less than 60 minutes, but may begin before or simultaneously with the aura.

References and further reading

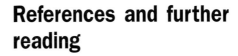

Becker WJ (1997) Migraine and oral contraceptives. *Can J Neurol Sci* **24**: 16–21.

Blau JN (1992) Migraine: theories of pathogenesis. *Lancet* **339**: 1202–7.

Blau JN, Thavapalan M (1988) Preventing migraine: a study of precipitating factors. *Headache* **28**: 481–3.

Bousser M-G, Conard J, Kittner S et al (2000) Recommendations on the risk of ischaemic stroke associated with use of combined oral contraceptives and hormone replacement therapy in women with migraine. *Cephalalgia* **20**: 155–6.

Carolei A, Marini C, De Matteis et al (1996) History of migraine and risk of cerebral ischaemia in young adults. *Lancet* **347**: 1503–6.

Chang CL, Donaghy M, Poulter N and WHO Collaborative Study of Cardiovascular Disease and Steroid Hormone Contraception (1999) Migraine and stroke in young women. *Br Med J* **318**: 13–18.

Collaborative Group for the Study of Stroke in Young Women (1975) Oral contraceptives and stroke in young women. *JAMA* **231**: 718–22.

De Lignières B, Vincens M, Mauvais-Jarvis P et al (1986) Prevention of menstrual migraine by percutaneous oestradiol. *Br Med J* **293**: 1540.

Drugs and Therapeutics Bulletin (1998). Managing migraine. **36**: 41–4.

Gross M, Barrie M, Bates D et al (1995) The efficacy of sumatriptan in menstrual migraine. *Eur J Neurol* **2**: 144–5.

Guillebaud J (2000) *Contraception Today* (4th edition). London: Martin Dunitz.

Headache Classification Committee of the International Headache Society (1988) Classification and diagnostic criteria for headache disorders, cranial neuralgias and facial pain. *Cephalalgia* **8** (Suppl 7): 1–96.

Keenan PA, Lindamer LA (1992) Non-migraine headache across the menstrual cycle in women with and without premenstrual syndrome. *Cephalalgia* **12**: 356–9.

Kubba A, Wilkinson C (1998) *Recommendations for clinical practice. Emergency Contraception.* London: Faculty of Family Planning and Reproductive Health Care of the Royal College of Obstetricians and Gynaecologists.

Lidegaard O (1993) Oral contraception and risk of a cerebral thromboembolic attack: results of a case-control study. *Br Med J* **306**: 956–63.

Lidegaard O (1995) Oral contraceptives, pregnancy and the risk of cerebral thromboembolism: the influence of diabetes, migraine and previous thrombotic disease. *Br J Obstet Gynaecol* **102**: 153–9.

MacGregor EA (1996) Menstrual migraine: towards a definition. *Cephalalgia* **16**: 11–21.

MacGregor EA (1997) Menstruation, sex hormones and migraine. *Neurolog Clin* **15**: 125–41.

MacGregor EA (1999) Estrogen replacement: a trigger for migraine aura? *Headache* **39**: 674–8.

MacGregor EA (1999a) *Managing migraine in primary care.* Oxford: Blackwell Science.

MacGregor EA (1999b) Effect of oral and transdermal oestrogen on migraine. *Cephalalgia* **19**: 124–5.

MacGregor EA (2000) Management of the menopause in women with migraine. *J Br Men Soc* **6**: 75–7.

MacGregor EA (2000) Women with migraine. In: Killick S (ed), *Contraception in Current Practice.* London: Martin Dunitz: 207–28.

MacGregor EA, Chia H, Vohrah RC, Wilkinson M (1990) Migraine and menstruation: a pilot study. *Cephalalgia* **10**: 305–10.

MacGregor EA, Guillebaud J (1998) Recommendations for clinical practice: combined oral contraceptives, migraine and ischaemic stroke. *Br J Fam Plan* **24**: 53–60.

MacGregor EA, Hackshaw A (2002) Prevention of migraine in the pill-free week of combined oral contraceptives using natural oestrogen supplements. *J Fam Plann Reprod Healthcare* **28**: 27–31.

Martins AD, Tanus SPC, Toledo LM, Viaira EE (1988) Treatment of nausea and vomiting of pregnancy with domperidone. *J Bras Ginecol* **98**: 65–9.

Massiou H, MacGregor EA (2000) Evolution and treatment of migraine with oral contraceptives. *Cephalalgia* **20**: 170–4.

Murray SC, Muse KN (1997) Effective treatment of severe menstrual migraine headaches with gonadotrophin-releasing hormone agonist and "add-back" therapy. *Fertil Steril* **67**: 390–3.

Nappi RE, Cagnacci A, Granella F et al (2001) Course of primary headaches during hormone replacement therapy. *Maturitas* **38**: 157–63.

Neri I, Granella F, Nappi R et al (1993) Characteristics of headache at menopause: a clinico-epidemiologic study. *Maturitas* **17**: 31–7.

Newman LC, Lipton RB, Lay CL, Solomon S (1998) A pilot study of oral sumatriptan as intermittent prophylaxis of menstruation-related migraine. *Neurology* **51**: 307–9.

Newman LC, Mannix LK, Landy S et al (2001) Naratriptan as short-term prophylaxis of menstrually associated migraine: a randomized double-blind, placebo-controlled study. *Headache* **41**: 248–56.

O'Brien PMS (1993) Helping women with pre menstrual syndrome. *Br Med J* **307**: 1471–5.

Olesen J, Tfelt-Hansen P, Welch KMA, eds (2000) *The Headaches*. Philadelphia: Lippincott, Williams and Wilkins.

Pradalier A Vincent D, Beaulieu PH et al (1994) Correlation between oestradiol plasma level and therapeutic effect on menstrual migraine. In: Rose FC (ed.), *New Advances in Headache Research*. London: Smith-Gordon: 129–32.

Rasmussen BK (1995) Epidemiology of headache. *Cephalalgia* **15**: 45–68.

Ratinahirana H, Darbois Y, Bousser MG (1990) Migraine and pregnancy: a prospective study in 703 women after delivery. *Neurology* **40**(suppl 1): 437.

Russell MB, Olesen J (1996) A nosographic analysis of the migraine aura in the general population. *Brain* **119**: 355–61.

Sances G, Martignoni E, Fioroni L et al (1990) Naproxen sodium in menstrual migraine prophylaxis: a double-blind placebo controlled study. *Headache* **30**: 705–9.

Silberstein SD, Lipton RB, Goadsby PJ (1998) *Headache in Clinical Practice*. Oxford: ISIS Medical Media.

Sillanpää M, Anttila P (1996) Increasing prevalence of headache in 7-year-old schoolchildren. *Headache* **36**: 466–70.

Smith R, Studd JWW (1993) *The Menopause and HRT*. London: Martin Dunitz.

Somerville BW (1971) The role of progesterone in menstrual migraine. *Neurology* **21**: 853–9.

Somerville BW (1972) The role of estradiol withdrawal in the etiology of menstrual migraine. *Neurology* **22**: 355–65.

Stein GS (1981) Headaches in the first post partum week and their relationship to migraine. *Headache* **21**: 201–5.

Steiner M, Yonkers K (1998) *Depression in women*. London: Martin Dunitz.

Stewart WF, Lipton RB, Chee et al (2000) Menstrual cycle and headache in a population sample of migraineurs. *Neurology* **55**: 1517–23.

Tzourio C, Tehindrazanarivelo A, Iglésias S et al (1995) Case-control study of migraine and risk of ischaemic stroke in young women. *Br Med J* **310**: 830–3.

Van Eijkeven MA, Christiaens GC, Geuze HJ et al (1992) Effects of mefenamic acid on menstrual haemostasis in essential menorrhagia. *Am J Obstet Gynecol* **166**: 1419–28.

Wall VR (1992) Breastfeeding and migraine headaches. *J Hum Lact* **8**: 209–12.

Wainscott G, Sullivan M, Volans GN, Wilkinson M (1978) The outcome of pregnancy in women suffering from migraine. *Postgrad Med J* **54**: 98–102.

Whitehead M, Godfree V (1992) *HRT: Your Questions Answered.* Edinburgh: Churchill Livingstone.

Wilkinson M, Williams K, Leyton M (1978) Observations on the treatment of an acute attack of migraine. *Res Clin Study Headache* 6: 141–6.

WHO Collaborative Study of Cardiovascular Disease and Steroid Hormone Contraception (1996) Ischaemic stroke and combined oral contraceptives: results of an international, multicentre, case-control study. *Lancet* 348: 498–505.

WHO (2000) Improving access to quality care in family planning (Second Edn). *Medical eligibility criteria for initiating and continuing use of contraceptive methods.* Geneva: WHO 1996.

Index

Schmidt

St. Louis Community College
at Meramec
Library